Diagnosing the Child, Diagnosing the Mother:
The Experience of Birth Mothers of Children Diagnosed
with Fetal Alcohol Spectrum Disorder

A DISSERTATION
SUBMITTED TO THE FACULTY OF THE GRADUATE SCHOOL
OF THE UNIVERSITY OF MINNESOTA

By

Diane Roselyn Monnens Anderson

IN PARTIAL FULFILLMENT OF THE REQUIREMENTS
FOR THE DEGREE OF
DOCTOR OF PHILOSOPHY

Dr. Jane Plihal, Advisor

January 2010

UMI Number: 3399779

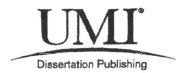

Dissertation Publishing

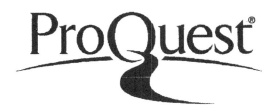

ProQuest LLC
789 East Eisenhower Parkway
P.O. Box 1346
Ann Arbor, MI 48106-1346

Acknowledgements

I would like to thank God for sustaining me during this educational adventure. I began my studies with the faith that He would see me through. With Him, all things are possible; He has brought me to success.

My family has shown unwavering support when I doubted myself, relentless pushing when I found many other things to distract me from my studying and writing, and an undying faith that I could meet my huge goal of completing a PhD. They learned to cook for themselves, work around and never touch my piles of books and papers, and accommodate my swinging emotions. I will be forever grateful for, and in awe of, their sacrifices.

Jane Plihal has been an advisor and mentor. She has been patient and supportive. She was intuitive about when she needed to stand back and let me struggle or push me to get the work done. She never expected less than my best.

I also wish to thank my examining committee: Susan Walker, Francis Lawrenz, and Ruth Thomas. Their thoughtful comments and questions encouraged me to think more deeply about my work.

I want to especially thank Sheila Moriarty and Nicole Bates-Childs for their encouragement and guidance, for commenting and editing, and especially for their commitment in helping me understand hermeneutic phenomenology and uncover the themes that they saw more clearly than I.

I have been privileged to work with great faculty in the University of Minnesota's Program in Occupational Therapy and the Department of Occupational Therapy at the College of St. Scholastica. They were convinced I could be successful in earning a PhD and their support and encouragement carried me through difficult times when I had no idea how I could possibly do my job and still complete coursework and writing this dissertation.

Finally, I am deeply grateful to the mothers who opened their hearts, bared their souls, and shared their pain in knowing they were the cause of their children's struggles. Their openness and honesty was amazing. Their stories were truly a gift they gave to me in the hopes that they could help other women.

i

Abstract

Fetal Alcohol Spectrum Disorder (FASD) is a constellation of physical, behavioral, emotional, social, and cognitive deficits caused solely by a mother drinking while pregnant. For every identified child there is a mother who comes to know she is the cause of her child's disabilities. How does she feel, think, and react when she comes to fully understand the FASD diagnosis? The purpose of this study was to describe the lived experience of birth mothers receiving the diagnosis of FASD for their child.

Hermeneutic phenomenological methodology was used to answer the research question. Nine birth mothers were interviewed about their experience. The interview transcripts were analyzed using van Manen's holistic examination and linguistic transformation until the themes of the experience were revealed. Hermeneutic interpretation was used to deepen the meanings uncovered in the analysis.

Five themes emerged from the analysis of the transcripts. The first theme, *something doesn't seem right with my child*, describes the sense of dread that something is wrong. Then the words are spoken, and the consequential meaning of the diagnosis shifts from child to mother in the theme *I can't believe this is happening to me*, and back to the child with the theme *I can't believe I've done this to my child*. The theme *I need you to see me, hear me, help me* reflects the experience of the mother with the health care provider who made the diagnosis. Finally, to the mother the receiving of the diagnosis is lifelong, reflected in the theme *I can't fix it; I can't make it better*.

The themes revealed in this study have implications for health care and education specialists. By deeply understanding and appreciating the mothers' experience we can better anticipate the kinds of supports they might need and the approaches from the diagnostics team that might be most useful to the mothers at the time of the diagnosis. We can empower the mothers and help them come to terms with their own experience so they are better able to meet the unique needs of their child with FASD.

Table of Contents

Chapter One: Inspiration for the Study

Angels Danced

I saw a greeting card with the words
"The Angels Danced on the Day you were Born."
and I wondered what kind of music was playing
as they danced for you.

Was it a woeful sad ballad that spoke of the
confusion, violence and addiction that surrounded your birth?
Was it a marching song that told of your persistence
and strength to overcome and conquer?
Was it a beautiful lullaby that helped you to sleep
in a world that was not very nurturing and soft?

Was there an orchestra full of trumpets and cymbals
majestically announcing the arrival of a special child of God?
Maybe the song had a wild rock beat,
the kind of song that you now love to dance to,
and maybe the angels twirled and giggled as they danced
much like you do now.

I wondered if they danced again
on the day you entered foster care.
Or the day we adopted you.
I know that I danced on that day.
I danced to your song
a song that only you can play,
a song that God allowed me to hear
but that not everybody hears yet.

Your daddy and I love to dance to your song
and we will keep inviting others to dance with us.

Your song is your gift to us
and we are blessed to be able to hear it.
It was your beautiful song that the angels heard that day,
wasn't it?
Keep playing, sweetheart.
They are still dancing!

(Fletcher, 2008; mother of a
child with FASD)

I've not always been interested in mothers and children. Motherhood was not something to which I aspired, and I approached it reluctantly and resentfully. In fact, my family and friends openly discouraged me from becoming a parent. I privately wonder at my metamorphosis to mother and grandmother. It seems to have just happened without my conscious will or self-direction. Part of my wonder is that I'm actually pretty successful in these roles. But in spite of my apparent success, I am plagued by my own beliefs that I can yet fail, that I am really not all that good at mothering, that things that I may have done as a younger person will still catch up with me and, more importantly, will affect my now grown children. One of those things I did as a younger person was to drink while pregnant. I was lucky. My son wasn't seriously impacted—he's a wonderful young man making a good life for himself and his family. It could have been so very different. It is my own history, reinforced by the career path I chose for myself and the experiences I've had with my clients, that has led me to this passion to more deeply understand the lived experiences of birth mothers of children diagnosed with Fetal Alcohol Spectrum Disorder (FASD).

Becoming Interested in FASD

I first became aware of Fetal Alcohol Spectrum Disorder while working as an occupational therapist in an early intervention program for children abused or neglected by their parents. Our focus was maintaining and strengthening the family unit, including working with parents in skills development and providing therapy to children to move them along their developmental continuum. However, much as we tried, there were some parents and some children who didn't seem to make progress. Out of my frustration with

2

what I saw as noncompliant mothers and ruined children, and wanting answers to how I could better work with them, I ventured back into higher education to pursue a degree in public health, with a specialty in maternal and child health.

As I searched for a master's thesis project, I was offered an opportunity to work with a small committee that was developing a working conference to address the Minnesota problem of Fetal Alcohol Syndrome. The intent of the conference was to bring together representatives across the state who were involved with prevention, intervention, research, and public policy related to FASD. The goal was to develop policy, establish a consistent research agenda, and collaborate on statewide initiatives for prevention, diagnosis, and intervention. My final task (and my thesis project) was to lead the conference participants in action planning on initiatives they committed to undertaking, then follow up after six months to determine how well those action plans were being met. But before the committee could address its intent and goal, we needed to fully understand that which we were planning to address. So began months of research into what was known about FASD.

What we knew about FASD back in the late 1980s was minimal. However, as I read and studied in preparation for the conference, I became aware that many of the children with whom I was working in the early intervention program likely had FASD. In retrospect, I believe many of the mothers probably also had FASD. Many were using or were at high risk for substance abuse, and often the violence in their homes was the result of alcohol and drugs. And as I thought even further back to my earliest clinical work, I began to understand that many of the youth with whom I had previously worked in locked adolescent psychiatric and chemical dependency units also likely had FASD. They were the youth who, no matter what we tried as a treatment approach, didn't seem to understand or make changes in their behaviors. They consistently remained a threat to their own safety and health. These youth grew up to be the parents I would later work with in the early intervention program. My interest in FASD gradually shifted from just doing what I needed to do and understanding enough to be successful on my thesis, to a passionate interest in prevention of and intervention with FASD. I wanted to positively impact the lives of children with FASD and work with women of childbearing age who were at risk of having children with FASD. Later, as I began to more fully appreciate the family systems models of care, my interests expanded to include mothers caring for these children.

Why This Study Now?

But are there really so many women delivering babies with FASD that a study such as mine is relevant? Clearly there are a number of women who drink when they are pregnant. We hear and see messages warning women not to drink if pregnant or could potentially become pregnant. Different prevalence rates for FASD have been reported, with rates ranging from 0.2-2.0 cases per 1,000 live births, depending on ascertainment methods (Abel, 1995; Center for Disease Control [CDC], 1993; May & Gossage, 2001). Lupton, Burd, and Harwood (2004) found that 40,000 persons are diagnosed with FASD each year. Still, they believe that 95% of children who have been exposed to alcohol prenatally go undiagnosed. For every child diagnosed with FASD, there is a mother who caused the disorder by drinking while pregnant. For every child who is diagnosed with

4

FASD, there is a mother who is carrying the knowledge that she caused the child's disabilities. How does a mother come to know about her child's diagnosis and disabilities? How does she feel, think, and react when she comes to fully understand the FASD diagnosis?

I currently work with 2 of Minnesota's 14 existing or developing FASD multi-disciplinary diagnostics teams. An intensive hours' long battery of assessments is followed by a meeting with the client's parents or caregivers. It is during this meeting that the diagnosis is shared and future planning begins. It is my experience that considerable time is spent in diagnostic team meetings on labeling the deficits and describing to the caregivers what the diagnosis of FASD means for their child, but there is little if any time spent in helping caregivers understand what the diagnosis means for them as caregivers. What is it like for the clients, and for the mothers, to hear the FASD diagnosis? How is this processed? Are they able to hear the recommendations, or are they just hearing the diagnosis?

I believe that many times the mothers are in shock and grief. The health care professionals give the diagnosis, then immediately begin talking about potential outcomes, recommendations and referrals, and long-term plans. I believe a mother is stuck in her grief and pain. She must be allowed her pain, but also helped to overcome it, and she needs to be empowered to be able to help her child. I want the child diagnosed, but I also want health care providers to recognize that there is a mother involved as well, and she needs to be considered.

Research Question

This is a qualitative inquiry into the experiences of birth mothers who have received a diagnosis of Fetal Alcohol Spectrum Disorder for their child. To deepen my understanding of mothers' experiences, my research question is "What is the lived experience for the birth mother of receiving a diagnosis of Fetal Alcohol Spectrum Disorder for her child?" From the perspective of hermeneutic phenomenology, I came to understand and formulate the research question, and conduct and analyze interviews about the women's lived experiences of being a birth mother at the time her child received the FASD diagnosis.

Chapter Two: Understanding Fetal Alcohol Spectrum Disorders

My Sister…My Friend, no one understands or has the capacity to feel and share your pain as another mother—another who has experienced the grief, guilt, and shame of giving birth to a child disabled by her own use of alcohol during pregnancy. We have been and will continue to be called negligent, cruel, irresponsible, heartless, and on occasion, even evil. We will be unjustly judged by our ethnicity or by our lifestyles. Some of us, less visible because of our social standing, educational achievements or bank account balances will be accorded "philosophical grace." Some of us have support from our extended family members; some of us are the only ones who "know" why our children are not like all the others. Nonetheless, each of us bears our own burden—publicly or privately—known to all, or unknown by anyone except ourselves. It doesn't matter whether we drank alcohol addictively, abusively or casually, with or without consequences, with or without the advice of our doctors, with or without our partners. We, you and I, and multitudes of other mothers throughout the ages have given birth to children with diminished potentials. It's a fact. And we grieve. (LaFever, 1995)

Linda LaFever is one voice among many. She is a mother, who, like hundreds of other mothers, inadvertently damaged her baby by drinking while she was pregnant. It wasn't intentional, but nonetheless the baby was damaged. And she, like those hundreds of other mothers, must live with the consequences of her behaviors—the damage she will see daily, and the emotions with which she will daily struggle. What must be the experience of knowing you are responsible for the pain and struggles your child will face for a lifetime? To know that there is nothing you can do to take that away? To be judged by others for your child's behaviors and disabilities?

What Is This Thing They Call FASD?

FASD has been a part of the human experience since the beginning of time. Ever since man learned to stomp grapes or ferment grains to create mind-altering drinks, there have been children born with FASD. The earliest references to FASD can be found in

Judges 13:7 of the Bible where an angel tells the mother of the prophet Sampson, "Behold, thou shalt conceive and bear a son and now drink no wine or strong drink."

As early as the 1700s, medical reports associated a woman's drinking with producing unhealthy children. During the gin epidemic in England (1714-1750), a letter to Parliament stated that gin was the cause of children needing custodial care, and medical reports warned of the dangers of alcohol on the growing fetus (Abel, 1990). By the middle of the 19th century, physicians in France were describing characteristics of Fetal Alcohol Syndrome (FAS), with research continuing until the time of prohibition when efforts to recognize and document the impact of alcohol on the fetus all but disappeared. In fact, post-prohibition brought a plethora of studies supporting the moderate use of alcohol to improve pregnancies. It wasn't until the 1970s that FAS again made an appearance in the medical journals (Abel).

Jones, Smith, Ulleland, and Streissguth (1973) first reported a relationship between maternal alcohol use during pregnancy and the resulting effects on the child. In a landmark study of eight children of alcoholic mothers, they found characteristics such as "fine motor dysfunction, including tremulousness, weak grasp, and/or poor eye/hand coordination, delayed gross motor performance, self-stimulating behaviors, and growth deficiencies" (pp. 1269-70). These researchers concluded that children born to alcoholic mothers had a characteristic pattern of physical anomalies, growth deficiency, and central nervous system (CNS) involvement. Jones and Smith (1973) called this disorder Fetal Alcohol Syndrome.

Streissguth and O'Malley (2000) later proposed the term Fetal Alcohol Spectrum Disorders (FASD) to include "individuals who manifest mild to severe disturbances of physical, behavioral, emotional, and/or social functioning attributable to in utero alcohol exposure" (p.178). Fetal Alcohol Spectrum Disorders (FASD) has since been used to include the diagnoses of Fetal Alcohol Syndrome (FAS), Fetal Alcohol Effects (FAE), Alcohol-Related Behavioral Disorder (ARBD), and Alcohol-related Neurodevelopmental Disorder (ARND) (Barr & Streissguth, 2001).

FASD is diagnosed only in persons whose mother drank while she was pregnant. Each year, up to 20% of U.S. women use alcohol during pregnancy whether or not she knows she is pregnant (Ebrahim et al., 1998). FASD is not always the result of a woman who is alcoholic or even one who drinks to excess; it can also happen to the baby of a teen mother who binged a couple times at weekend parties. And one woman can drink heavily and have good birth outcomes while the next woman can drink only on occasion and deliver a child with FASD. The fact is we just don't know how much alcohol is damaging to the fetus, why two mothers can have the same drinking patterns and one has a child with FASD while the other doesn't, or why one baby is resilient to the damage while another has a great number of disabilities.

Currently, women comprise the fastest growing segment of the alcohol abusing population (National Council on Alcoholism and Drug Dependence [NCADD], 2002), and their alcohol use problems impact our society not just because of the numbers of women involved in unhealthy drinking with all of its consequences but also because of the potential of these women to bear children who have a Fetal Alcohol Spectrum

Disorder. According to the 2003 National Survey on Drug Use and Health (NSDUH), an estimated 5.9% of women aged 18 or older met criteria for abuse of, or dependence on, alcohol or an illicit drug in the past year (Department of Health and Human Services [DHHS], 2004a).

Birth defects related to prenatal alcohol exposure can occur in the first 3 to 8 weeks of pregnancy (DHHS, 2004c). According to the results of the 1999 and 2000 National Household Survey on Drug Abuse (NHSDA), pregnant women in their first trimester were more likely to report alcohol use than women whose pregnancies were more advanced (DHHS). It's clear that many women may be putting their child at risk for life-long disabilities by drinking before they may even know they are pregnant. There is also a high likelihood that a woman could become pregnant, not know she is pregnant, and continue to drink during the first weeks or months of that pregnancy, putting her unborn child at risk of FASD.

Alcohol and Women

If a woman knows drinking alcohol can damage her unborn child, why would she drink when she is pregnant? Or could potentially become pregnant? Why would she purposefully put her baby at risk of the long-term deficits associated with FASD? Society challenges mothers-to-be to make the right choices, using the latest research to tell them all about healthy pregnancy care and optimal child-rearing practices. Health care professionals, families, and friends also don't hesitate to offer advice. Part of this advice is a pervasive message not to drink when pregnant. We even see it on liquor bottles, signs in establishments that sell or serve liquor, in the bathrooms of restaurants, and on bus sides and billboards. However, there is a stronger societal message that using alcohol is cool, sophisticated, and even healthy. Often the medical profession delivers mixed messages to women. Frequently doctors tell women it's okay to drink. One should, after all, have a glass of red wine daily to protect one's heart, or to have a healthy and relaxed pregnancy. In their misunderstanding, women drink—for many reasons.

Both men and women drink, of course. But the relationship women have with alcohol is different from that of men. Circumstances in women's lives are different from those of men. This is reflected in the women's experience of substance use problems. Women's substance use problems are more stigmatized and less likely to be acknowledged than men's. Women who drink excessively are seen as deviant and their behavior is socially determined to be irresponsible (Reed, 1987). Because their drinking behavior is not considered "normal," women are further stigmatized with labels. When the labeling process occurs, society starts to isolate this group of women from mainstream society. This can severely limit a woman's ability to fully participate in the everyday life of society, such as holding a job, having a home, getting access to any needed services, and enjoying mutually supportive relationships with family and friends (Reed).

Women with substance use problems often have fewer resources (e.g., employment, education, and income) than men, are more likely to be living with a partner with a substance use problem, and are more likely to have responsibility for the care of dependent children, making the social stigmatizing process that much more difficult to face (DHHS, 2006). There is a sense of shame and guilt associated with the drinking

11

behavior. How much greater is that shame and guilt when the deviant and irresponsible behavior causes damage to her own child?

What is the experience, then, of having a child impacted by FASD caused by drinking before the woman even knew she was pregnant? What must it mean for mothers to drink even though they might know it's not healthy for their baby? And how must they feel when they deliver a damaged baby caused by doing something they had been warned not to do, or about which they had been given inaccurate information? Who is to blame? The doctor who gave an inaccurate message? Society for its message that drinking is socially accepted behavior, even for pregnant women? The mother who did the bad thing, purposefully or inadvertently? Too often, I believe it's the woman who bears the brunt of judgment for damaging her child.

Labeling the Disorder

A mother drinks; a baby can be born damaged. This damage is visible to all. A diagnosis of FASD is made based on four criteria. First, babies with FASD have distinctive facial features (short palpebral fissures making their eyes look wide-spread, a flattened philtrum or groove under the nose, and a thin upper lip). Second, they might have both height and weight deficiencies, and might have structural damage to their bodies. Whatever is developing in utero at the time of the alcohol insult may be damaged. The brain and central nervous system is particularly vulnerable; the third criterion, brain and central nervous system defects, result in lifelong learning disabilities and emotional and behavioral disorders. The alcohol related changes in the brain might be present even in babies whose appearance and growth are not affected. Finally, unique to diagnosing

12

FASD is the fact that maternal alcohol use during pregnancy must be identified either by the mother admitting to drinking when pregnant, or by someone who has observed her drinking and is willing to provide that evidence (CDC, 2005). This is especially critical if the child doesn't demonstrate the typical FASD facial features. FASD is, in fact, a diagnosis where the culpability of the mother must be made blatantly obvious. The mother must acknowledge her behavior, and take responsibility for damaging her child.

What does it mean to the mother to have her child diagnosed with FASD? To be labeled as something? The *Oxford English Dictionary* (2006) defines diagnosis as the decision or opinion resulting from investigating the facts or nature of something. It is the recognition and identification of something by examination or investigation. It is the clinical facts stripped of emotions. It is the cause and effect, the outcomes of past behaviors, a breakdown of systems, the labeling of a dysfunction that sets this diagnosed person apart from others. A diagnosis may come to define the child to whom it is attached.

A diagnosis is external—it is applied to a child. We mark a child with FASD as damaged. We can say the child will be forever set apart by facial features, the behaviors that are shown, and the dysfunction manifested in school and in the community. But in giving the diagnosis of FASD, we also apply a diagnosis to the mother. As we mark that child, we mark the mother, labeling her for what she has done in the past and what she has inflicted on her child. We make her accountable.

> We live in a computerized society, one in which we are warned not to fold, spindle, or mutilate. But mothers and children are repeatedly folded, spindled, and mutilated in an effort to make them fit into institutions and ideas designed to serve large numbers of people rather than individuals. When dealing

with numbers it is inevitable that a hypothetical norm becomes the standard against which everyone is measured. Deviations from this norm present a problem, because they require special thought and attention. As a result, it is automatically bad not to conform to the norm. Differences are undesirable. It is not "normal" to be different. This is the message given to mothers about their children and themselves. Diversity and differences in development are not readily tolerated by those whose function it is to serve the needs of children, but the onus is shifted to the child and by implication to the mother. The idea is that if the child doesn't fit in, there is something wrong with the child. If there is something wrong with the child, something also must be wrong with the mother. (Heffner, 1978, pp. 131-132)

When a diagnosis of FASD is given to a child, the child and the mother are told that the child will forever be different. He is damaged and unfixable. He will forever be *not normal* in a society that not only sets the definition of normal and different, but also does not readily tolerate those differences. Messages are given to the mothers about their children and about themselves. If something is wrong with the child, we are quick to blame the mother. Considered in context, we can amplify that judgment by the fact that FASD is caused by the mother. She becomes bad, criminal, uncaring, or abusive. Herein lays a debate that has been a part of FASD since it was first diagnosed. Why do we need to label the child?

For years there has been controversy over the need to attach a label to the child with FASD. Opponents to labeling talk about the secondary victimization of the mother who must make her behaviors known to all. They talk about the stigma the mother feels because she has damaged her child, and the stigma society places on her as a person who is chemically dependent. She is automatically assumed to be irresponsible, lacking in emotional stability, and lacking in parenting ability. The opponents to labeling also talk about the stigma the child feels at being marked the product of a bad mother. And they cite the literature that discusses the imbalance of diagnosis based on race and socio-economic status. So the question again is why do we need to attach a label to a child, especially a label that implicates a mother's behaviors? What is the value to the mother of seeking a diagnosis for her child? Why would she look for a name for what has happened to her baby if she knows she will be judged?

A diagnosis—a label—is crucial to ensure that the child qualifies for early intervention services and that appropriate behavioral and environmental management strategies are put in place to prevent some of the long-term, secondary disabilities commonly seen in young people with FASD. The system needs the diagnosis to justify providing services. With a diagnosis, there is a sense of hidden shame, yet there is also open shame—you must acknowledge your bad behavior to get the services your child needs. You're damned if you do, damned if you don't get that label for your child.

Good Mother-Bad Mother

As a mother, I've anxiously waited for a child to reach a milestone, secretly (and not so secretly) comparing my children to nieces and nephews and to others' children in the parks, schools, stores, and at church. I've wondered where I failed as a mother when one of my children did something wrong or didn't do what I expected or wanted. According to Heffner (1978) in her book *Mothering: The Emotional Experience of Motherhood after Freud and Feminism*, mothers often create "bad mom" messages for themselves or perceive them in what others say. She writes that a woman's success as a mother is often measured (by others as well as the mother herself) by the behaviors and successes of the child. I know in my head that what I do or say will most likely not scar my children for life, but my heart says differently. I fear, and am quite sure, that I'm being judged by others for my mothering abilities because of the ways my children chose to live their lives. I know that I'm no different from any other mother. My children are healthy and doing well, for the most part. I had uneventful and healthy pregnancies. I tried to do everything "right," based on the many books I read. I tried to follow the directions of my doctor and nurses. But I drank while pregnant. My doctor suggested that a drink a day would help calm me; she believed "a calm mother is a better mother" and apparently didn't know about FASD. I was lucky—or better said, my child was lucky. That I drank while pregnant is a fact I chose not to share with family or friends, anticipating that my son's behaviors would be judged even more harshly than they were. Still I wonder how my perceptions of others' reactions to me would be different if this mistake, done purposeful out of ignorance and error, had impacted the health and well-being of my son. How would I be judged and have my mothering abilities questioned by others?

To be a mother is to be vulnerable to judgment. There are good mothers; there are bad mothers. What does it mean to be a good mother? Is it even something mothers can attain? If society defines a good mother, and sanctions a bad mother, what does this mean for women who have a child diagnosed with FASD? Clearly they have failed the good mother test.

By most standards, a good mother is caring, dedicated, and selfless, providing for her family's needs and desires. She is loving and caring, patient above all else, calm and relaxed, and a good listener. She takes care of the maintenance tasks of rearing a child, as well as the tasks of maintaining a home (Brown & Smith, 1997; Elkins, 1991; Larson, 2000; Phoenix & Woollett, 1991). The stereotype of the perfect mother is one who devotes all her time and energy to caring for her children, especially the child with disabilities. If she needs to ask for assistance, if she needs help to care for that child with disabilities, she fears this will be interpreted as not loving the child enough—being a bad mother (Elkins; Larson, 2000). Her fears are often substantiated by others. Phoenix and Woollett (1991) write that "the tasks of mothering are socially proscribed so that many mothers learn that it is extremely difficult to mother well" (p. 13). Mothers quickly label themselves as bad if they don't meet societal expectations in a society that gives little room for parenting differently.

Following an examination of texts on infant and child care, Marshall (1991) delineated the many myths of good mothering. Unfortunately, these myths have been accepted by mothers across generations, and they cause us to judge ourselves as mothers and to judge the other mothers in our lives. According to Marshall's list of myths, a good mother finds mothering to be the most fulfilling, exciting, and creative occupation she could possibly have. A good mother loves her child immediately and unconditionally. Even if that love is not immediate, it will always come to be and will always be total. As mothers, we are led to believe that maternal love is a remembrance of the unconditional and total love of our own mothers, because of course all good mothers are loving and caring people. But even though a good and loving mother is the product of another good and loving mother, we accept the myth that professionals know best how to raise a child. Because the professionals are assumed to know best, a good mother does not rely on the experiences of mothers from past generations. (Other women helping women is unacceptable). A modern, informed, and concerned—that is good—mother relies on the experts. We are asked to believe that children must be brought up in a two-parent family (father and mother) to be healthy and whole. A single mother is a bad mother. A mother is responsible for stimulating and facilitating her child's development by providing a safe environment, monitoring normal development, and looking out for abnormalities. The disability must be the fault of a bad mother. Finally, if the pressure of parenting an infant is not enough, a myth prevails that a mother must know that her early relationship with her child impacts the child's future relationships with the child's partner, as well as the child's intellectual growth, emotional depth, and ability to avoid delinquent behavior. It is so easy to be bad!

Professional literature, even today, continues to blame parents, especially mothers, for the problems of their children. Unsuccessful mothers are isolated, subject to criticism and blame (Elkins, 1991; Klein, 1993). Even as much as the literature and professionals criticize and blame her, so too does the mother judge herself if she is unable to meet the criteria of good mothering.

To be a good mother is to be in a good relationship with the child, one where the child's needs are met with understanding and care, and where the mother has a sense of self and of purpose (Brown & Small, 1997). There is a commitment of mother to child that belongs only between them (Brown & Small). Imagine the pain of the mother who does not immediately bond with her baby, something that frequently happens with infants with disabilities such as those seen with FASD. Generations of mothers before her have apparently been able to do the simplest of mothering tasks—loving her child and being loved in return. But does the mother of a child with FASD have the right to expect this when she apparently didn't love her unborn child enough not to drink? Leavitt (2006) writes, "He didn't seem to like me, and I hadn't a clue what to do about it other than to sometimes, to my great shame and bewilderment, not like him back. The great myth is that mother love comes instantly, as natural as breathing" (p. 44). The mother of a child with disabilities often struggles to feel love for a child and is shamed by her feelings of fear, guilt, and maybe disgust. Multiply that shame for the mother who knows she caused her child's disability, the very disability that interferes with this early love relationship between mother and baby.

A common belief is that women are happiest as mothers, and even their successes in life are associated with nurturing and mothering. Motherhood is seen as nature's intention for women, and creative activity is just a substitution for childbearing and nurturing; women would be restless and miserable without motherhood (Elkins, 1991). A good mother, then, is one who welcomes a baby into her life, willingly, longingly, and with no regrets. She has "a 'passion for maternity.' It manifests itself instinctively in doing the right thing, despite criticism and advice, well-meaning or otherwise" (Elkins, 1991, p. 115). A woman cannot move reluctantly or accidently into motherhood and still be considered a good mother.

"Society expects women to be nurturers, caretakers of personal relationships, the self-sacrificers; and to remain on the periphery of the larger power structure" (Elkins, 1991, p. 111). Through their work with welfare policy and women, Reid, Greaves, and

Poole (2008) found that the definition of a good mother was one who does not allow herself or her children to come to public attention. The child "turns out right" by being brought up in "the right circumstances," however that is defined by society. According to these authors, a mother calls the attention of the welfare system to herself if she is raising her child alone, is a teen mother or older mother, lives in poverty, lives in an environment of drug or alcohol use, or is a mother who works. But this doesn't account for the impact on mothers of society or social services systems. The "system" often defines mothers as bad because they are victims of their society. The poor mother, the teen mother, or the mother who must work needs to accept aid, and for that she is labeled. The mother who tries to reach out for help with a drug or alcohol problem risks being labeled as bad and deviant and having her children removed from her care (Reid, Greaves, & Poole). The mother of a child with FASD falls into many of these categories of badness. The difference between a good and a bad mother is sometimes the difference between middle and lower class. A case in point is that the child of a lower class mother is more quickly identified as FASD than the child of a middle or upper class woman.

Is a mother always good or always bad? In the interviews done by Brown and Small (1997), mothers were unable to straddle the good-bad dichotomy of mothering. If they could not be "good," in all of its many descriptors, they felt they were "bad." There was not partway; a mother couldn't see herself as sometimes good, sometimes not so good. Often times this dichotomy that mothers feel is reinforced by the public, by public policy, and by health care providers and education specialists. A mother once labeled as a mother of a child with FASD identifies herself, and is identified by others, as forever bad.

I drank when I was pregnant. I didn't know—back in the early '80s not many people knew about FAS. I didn't know drinking could hurt your baby. Back then, and still today, doctors are telling pregnant women it's OK to drink just a little. "It'll calm you. Calm moms have easier pregnancies. And happier babies." My son is in his 20's. He's got a good job, bought a house. I'm so very proud of what he is accomplishing. He's also a recovering alcoholic, barely passed high school, got in lots of trouble that sometimes involved the police. To this day, if I don't hear from him for a while I wonder if he's in trouble and doesn't want to worry me. And when the phone rings and I hear "mama" (he calls me mama when he's hurting or in trouble), my heart sinks. Did I cause this? Is it my fault he has to struggle so much in life?

The incident that sticks out the most in my mind happened when he 14. He was so overwhelmed with frustration at school. He wasn't "getting it," and teachers kept pushing and telling him he wasn't trying. He WAS trying. He's very smart—high IQ, people smart. But he can't concentrate; he's very distractible, and school just doesn't come easy. Well, after a particularly tough day, he came home, took a baseball bat, and smashed out the windows of all the cars in the parking lot behind our house. Then walked through the snow to our back door. No doubt in anyone's mind who had done the damage. I think that was the same week he threatened suicide. The same year I found where he had planted his marijuana and discovered how much he was drinking. The year he was in and out of treatment for alcohol use. The year he ran away weekend after weekend. It was a tough year, both for him and for me. We would have 5 more years of tough times; times when the phone would ring, and if he wasn't home, I would immediately feel my stomach turn and my heart ache, thinking—knowing— he was in trouble yet again. (Dolores, personal communication, June 18, 2006)

Mothers are protectors. From the moment a pregnancy is known, we believe mothers are to be protectors and teachers. A mother's concern is to first and foremost make sure her unborn child is safe and healthy, loved and cared for. She is to care for that child even above her own life (Barnard & Martell, 1995). What does it mean, then, for a mother to be the cause of her child's disabilities and suffering?

Society has the perspective that if a child is damaged, acts out, or shows emotional or behavioral problems, then the parents—the mother—is to be blamed. We look at parents to control behavior, to be responsible for their children. Some badness is to be expected of children, but what about the behavior of a child with FASD? Often above and beyond what a typical acting out child demonstrates, the behaviors of children with FASD are excessive in their intensity and duration. Society sits in judgment of the mother who can't teach or control her child. How is a mother to respond to such judgment? What must that be like for her to not only deal with the behaviors, and the judgments, but to also know that she is the cause?

This study explores more deeply the experiences of birth mothers of receiving the diagnosis of FASD for their child, of getting a label that tells the world that she was the sole cause of her child's life-long disability.

Chapter Three: Methodology and Method

The fundamental model of this approach is textual reflection on the lived experiences and practical actions of everyday life with the intent to increase one's thoughtfulness and practical resourcefulness or tact. Phenomenology describes how one orients to lived experience, hermeneutics describes how one interprets the "texts" of life. (van Manen, 1997, p. 4)

Choosing Phenomenology

The purpose of this study, understanding the lived experience of birth mothers of children receiving an FASD diagnosis, cannot be achieved by quantitatively surveying women about their opinions, or tallying common reactions from a checklist. A phenomenological approach allowed me to conduct empathetic interviewing to obtain a text of the women's experience. Active and reflective examination of this text and hermeneutic interpretation allowed me to deepen my understanding of the experience of birth mothers to reach what van Manen (1997) calls the essence, that is, when "the description reawakens or shows us the lived quality and significance of the experience in a fuller and deeper manner" (p. 10). This chapter further discusses the philosophical influences underpinning my research and describes the methods I used to answer my research question.

Philosophical Influences

Phenomenology defined. Phenomenology is the study of descriptions or structures of consciousness about an experience to find its essential or fundamental experienced meaning. It begins in a person's lifeworld or natural attitude and "aims at making explicit and seeking universal meaning" (van Manen, 1997, p. 19). We are to go to the things themselves, and allow them to show themselves to us (Husserl, 1907/1964).

Phenomenology requires that we turn to the thing that is to be studied, and that we take an open stance to what meaning the thing holds. To be open is to allow the phenomenon to present itself to us as it is and to intuit the essential meaning of the phenomenon, free of our beliefs of fact or causality (Husserl).

The things we want to understand, the phenomena, are defined by Husserl (1907/ 1964) as "appearance and that which appears" (p. 11). A phenomenon is and a phenomenon presents itself. Similarly, Heidegger (1927/1962) suggested that "we must keep in mind that the expression 'phenomenon' signifies that which shows itself in itself, the manifest" (p. 51).

Intentionality. A central concept of phenomenology is the idea of intentionality (Dahlberg, Drew, & Nyström, 2001). The principle of intentionality, as defined by van Manen (1997), is the "inseparable connection to the world. To know the world is to be in the world in a certain way. [It's] the intentional act of attaching ourselves to the world" (p. 5). What we experience has meaning to us, and we carry that meaning to later experiences. Further, as we experience something, we extend what is immediately accessible and present to us so that what we are experiencing, we perceive to be complete. We fill in the blanks and add to that experience based on our past experiences.

Husserl (1907/1964) defined intentionality as the directed awareness of a person toward objects or events. We understand the meaning of objects or events because of our relationship with them. Merleau-Ponty refers to intentionality as consciousness. "We are caught up in the world and we do not succeed in extricating ourselves from it in order to achieve consciousness of the world" (Merleau-Ponty, 1945/1962, p. 5). We cannot reflect on an experience as we experience it. We can only reflect in hindsight. We also cannot reflect on something until we have been made aware of it. When we are conscious of the object or event, we can give it meaning.

Gadamer (1960/1975) believed the intent of phenomenology is not to understand how something is, but to understand how something has become. According to Giorgi (1997), phenomenology "doesn't automatically want to say that something 'is', but it wants to understand what motivates a conscious creature to say that something 'is.' Thus, it has to begin at a more fundamental place, where there is 'presence' but not yet that type of presence to which one attributes 'existence'" (p. 239). Fink (1966/1972) defines phenomenology as "careful description and intuition which establishes laws of essences, which is applicable to any and every entity" (p. 23). So the goal of phenomenology is to describe, synthesize, and transform experiences until one arrives at the fundamental meaning of the experience.

Natural attitude and lifeworld. Husserl (1907/1964) believed that we all exist in what he refers to as the natural attitude, where we accept all of our experiences without reflection and with the attitude that everyone experiences as we do. When we are in the natural attitude, we accept that which appears to be the most obvious and don't look for other possible understandings. It is as it appears to be; deeper meaning is hidden (Dahlberg, Drew, & Nyström, 2001).

The natural attitude is our way of being in the world; our lifeworld is our way of experiencing the world. Husserl (1907/1964) described lifeworld (i.e., natural thinking) as the "original, pre-reflective, pre-theoretical attitude." It is "life as we experience it pre-reflectively rather than as we conceptualize, categorize, or reflect on it" (Husserl, p. 15).

Gadamer, (1960/1975) used the term lifeworld to describe "the world in which we are

immersed in the natural attitude that never becomes an object as such for us, but that

represents the pregiven basis of all experience" (pp. 246-247). Merleau-Ponty

(1945/1962) believed this lifeworld to be the basis of knowledge, and the way in which

we relate to and interact with the world.

Heidegger (1927/1962) believed that phenomena lie undiscovered, buried over, or

disguised. He defined phenomenology as the search for that thing that is hidden or does

not show itself; or for that thing that has become forgotten or its meaning is not

questioned. Phenomenological investigation begins with deeply questioning a lifeworld

phenomenon to bring to light its essential nature and meaning. Husserl (1907/1964)

called this the search for the: objectivity of essences" (p. 6), the seeing of something in its

pure self. These pure self or fundamental meanings are the essence (or eidos) of the

experience.

The essence of an experience is what is, and what is given; it is "the constitution,

the intrinsic character" (p. 24) of the experience. It makes the phenomenon what it is.

Without it, the phenomenon would not exist. An essence has "a meaning [that] remains

constant in spite of factual variation in the experience of its particular manifestations"

(Polkinghorne, 1989, p. 42). A number of people can experience the same phenomenon

in a variety of contexts and the essential meaning—the eidos—of these experiences

remains constant. Phenomenological investigation is turning "to the things themselves"

(Heidegger, 1927/1962, p. 50) to enable a phenomenologist to see how the phenomenon is being fully experienced, to look for the essence of it, or that which makes the experience what it is, no matter who experiences it or the context in which it is experienced. According to Merleau-Ponty (1945/1962), finding the fundamental meaning of an experience is "truth in itself in which the reason underlying all appearances is to be found" (p. 54). There is, in the belief of these philosophers, a universal meaning underlying the many manifestations of a common experience.

In our search for the essence of an experience, we bring to our phenomenological questioning preconceived ideas, assumptions, and our own personal belief that what we experienced is the way that it is for everyone else. We conclude that the phenomenon we are experiencing exists and that it is real. Heidegger (1927/1964) stated that "the very fact that we already live in an understanding of Being and that the meaning of Being is still veiled in darkness proves that it is necessary in principle to raise the question again" (p. 23). Phenomenological questioning provokes a response or recognition of the same or a similar personal experience. The trick to phenomenological questioning is to be in conversation with a research participant, to question deeply, to keep the interviewee focused, yet keep our own personal experiences of the phenomenon from prejudicing or leading what is being revealed (van Manen, 1976).

Openness in phenomenological investigation is the ability to *be with* the phenomenon without imposing pre-understanding, prejudices, and biases to the questioning or the understanding of that phenomenon. To be open includes being in a reduction stance, which is the act of suspending all beliefs about the object of the study.

Openness is necessary in the questioning, in transforming the text, and finally in coming to understand the meaning of the phenomenon.

Reduction. We live in the world as we understand it, and the world gives us our perceptions of who we are and what we do. We accept what we believe to be; we have constructed our meanings of the world as we are a part of that world. Phenomenological reduction demands that we reflect on the natural world, that we no longer accept that which we have always believed to be. We set aside our own knowledge of theories related to the natural world phenomenon to be open to the essence of what is underneath the natural world. Husserl (1907/1964) invented the technique of reduction as a means to look closely at the presence of something, without saying that it, in fact, exists. He described two levels of reduction—phenomenological reduction and eidetic reduction.

The phenomenological reduction is Husserl's response to scientific inquiry, and the claim that it is an exact science (Husserl, 1913/1931). In scientific inquiry, the scientist accepts without question the natural world and the things of the natural world. Husserl believed that this was inadequate because there was no grounding in "a strictly scientific philosophy" (p. 96). He saw that the natural world was composed of hypotheses, scientific conceptions, and psychological influences that had not been subject to critical examination but were accepted as givens. In his mind, inquiry needed to start at the pure world, with "a scientific essential knowledge of consciousness, toward that which consciousness itself 'is' according to its essence in all its distinguishable forms" (p. 114). To get to the pure world, there needed to be a stripping away of the natural world until the "things themselves" were exposed. He refers to this stripping away as phenomenological reduction.

According to Husserl (1907/1964), we look at objects in terms of our self; we perceive the object as it is given and sensed. These perceptions are transcendent—phenomenological reduction removes anything transcendent, to get to the pure phenomenon "which exhibits its intrinsic (immanent) essence" (p. 35). He believed that phenomenological reduction eliminates both the philosophical and the pre-givenness of the lifeworld, so a researcher can achieve transcendentiality (a stepping out of and away from the natural attitude).

Phenomenological reduction, as Husserl conceived it, consists of two "moments" that are in interplay (Husserl, 1907/1964). The first moment, the epoché, is that moment where we no longer accept the world as it appears to be (known as the pre-critical or human immanence). It's not that we deny that the world exists as we had always thought, but that we suspend those beliefs to be able to look more reflectively at something we want to more deeply understand (Cogan, 2006; Scott, 2003). In the second moment, the reduction proper, we come to recognize that we have accepted our acceptance of the lifeworld in the first place. "Epoché is the 'moment' in which we abandon the acceptedness of the world that holds us captive and the reduction proper indicates the 'moment' in which we come to the transcendental insight that the acceptedness of the world *is* an acceptedness and not an absolute. The structure of the phenomenological reduction has belonging to it the human I standing in the natural attitude, the transcendental constituting I, and the transcendental phenomenologizing I [onlooker]"

(Cogan, p. 12). It's through these two moments of the phenomenological reduction that we are able to come to understand the meaning of a phenomenon.

Phenomenological reduction has been likened to a spiritual awakening and a transformation of thinking. Fink (1966/1972) speaks of the rigor of the act of phenomenological reduction as,

> The philosophical 'unchaining,' the tearing oneself free from the power of one's naïve submission to the world, the stepping-forth from out of that familiarity with entities which always provides us with security, in one word, the phenomenological epoché, is anything but a noncommittal, 'merely' theoretical, intellectual act; it is rather a spiritual movement of one's self *encompassing* the *entire man* and, as an attack upon the 'state-of-motionlessness' supporting us in our depths, the pain of a *fundamental transformation down to our roots.* (p. 9)

The second level of phenomenological reduction, the eidetic reduction (Husserl, 1907/1964), is where we come to understand that what we had accepted about our natural world, is just that—an unquestioned acceptance that a constructed belief is an absolute, when in reality it is not. In eidetic reduction we look past the lived experience itself to find the essence or eidos of that experience. We "make the pure essence of perception give itself to our pure intuition" (p. xvii). Here intuition can be defined as ordinary ways of knowing (Giorgi, 1997). Husserl refers to this as the genuine immanence of the object, that "which presents only itself adequately and nothing outside itself" (p. 3), and excludes anything that is transcendent immanence (anything else). It was not enough to only understand my natural attitude toward the women in my study. It was also not acceptable to put my personally held beliefs onto the meaning the women had of their experience. I needed to allow the essence of the women's experience to reveal itself through unbiased listening, intuition, imaginative variation, and deep reflection.

Finally, if we are to arrive at the essence of a thing (a phenomenon), we must constitute its meaning (Husserl, 1907/1964). The concept of constitution is "an act which makes the object present" until we come to "grasp the meaning of the absolute given, the absolute clarity of the given, which excludes every meaningful doubt, in a word, to grasp the absolutely 'seeing' evidence which gets hold of itself" (p. 7). It is through eidetic reduction that we begin to see themes and patterns of meaning. Having suspended my beliefs (my natural attitude) about the women in my study, I used phenomenological and eidetic reduction to open myself to the meaning of their experiences, free from my preconceptions. I wanted to listen to their stories until the meaning of the experiences *to them* was revealed to me. To reach the essence of the women's experience I had to "trace all forms of giveness [of the experience] and all correlations and conduct an elucidatory analysis" (p. 10).

Bracketing. Husserl (1907/1964) uses the term transcendental subjectivity to define a further reduction where the researcher brackets out the self to get rid of inductive or deductive conclusions, everything that is not pure evidence or essence, to be left with "the meaning of the absolute given, the absolute clarity of the given…to grasp the absolute 'seeing' evidence which gets hold of itself" (p. 7). Merleau-Ponty (1964/1968) refers to this as hyper-reflection, and of the phenomenon, states that one is not to "lose sight of the brute things and the brute perception," but to reflect on the "transcendence of the world as transcendence" (p. 38) in order to reach some universal truth that has not yet been put to words. One must not be limited to what is deduced from what is experienced in the senses, but the researcher must strip away (transcend) the sense experience to get to the pure phenomenon. van Manen (2002) suggests that to achieve phenomenological reduction, one needs to "bracket all knowledge, all theory or theoretical meaning, all belief in what is real, and aim at evoking concreteness or living meaning" (p. 1). All of these theoretical or scientific bits of knowledge abstract the meaning of the phenomenon, preventing us from seeing the essence of the thing as it exists. There is a danger that if I as a phenomenologist do not first bring to my conscious awareness my pre-understandings of an experience, through reduction and bracketing, these pre-understandings will go unnoticed and affect the meaning of what is being revealed to me by my informants. In the words of Merleau-Ponty (1964/1968), "reflection [on a perception or phenomenon] is not to presume upon what it finds and condemn itself to putting into the things what it will then pretend to find in them, it must suspend the faith in the world only so as to see it, only so as to read in it the route it has followed in becoming" (p. 38). Reflection is needed so that I don't inadvertently search for my meanings—my personal prejudices—in the phenomenon being interpreted, but that I allow the meanings to reveal themselves through the pre-reflective descriptions of my informants.

Openness. Critical to hermeneutic phenomenology is openness to the phenomenon (Dahlberg, Drew, & Nyström, 2001). This is the idea that the world can show itself to us. In phenomenological research, we move into the text or observation or experience expecting to find something new. We remain open to the unexpected new understanding (Dahlberg, Drew, & Nyström). Openness is an attitude of discovery. To be open is to wait for the essential meaning of the phenomenon to be revealed to us.

"The hermeneutic task becomes of itself a questioning of things" (Gadamer 1960/1975, p. 238). We remain open and interested in understanding. Because we come to the situation interested, we come with some sense of the meaning of the experience; we have a prejudice toward the meaning. But because we are interested and open to both the research situation and to ourselves, we are willing to challenge our prejudices with different meanings and assimilate those meanings into a new sense of what is (Dahlberg, Drew, & Nyström, 2001). The results of our investigation and analysis, as phenomologists, must come from the data and not from prejudices and pre-understandings (Gadamer, trans. 1976) or pre-structures and implicit knowledge (Merleau-Ponty, 1945/1962). As such, it's critical that we are self-aware so that our prejudices or pre-structures don't cause us to anticipate meanings.

In my study, I needed to wait for the meaning of the experience of receiving a diagnosis for a child to make itself known to me through the words of the mothers. I needed to remain open to their experiences in spite of my own similar personal experiences. Remaining open was critical to avoid closing off discovery before the essential meaning of the mothers' experiences was revealed.

Hermeneutics. Hermeneutics is defined by the *Oxford Old English Dictionary* (2006) as the art or science of interpretation, especially of scripture. The hermeneutic method goes beyond exposition or explanation to find the profound and hidden meaning of objects, texts, or events. It is used to increase knowledge by describing, interpreting, and understanding experiences.

Phenomena show themselves to us, and it is hermeneutic interpretation (Gadamer, 1960/1975) that allows us to unravel their meaning. How we understand the world is based on how we interpret it. New experiences build on history and tradition (Weinsheimer, 1985). We come to understand by being-in-the-world, as it is influenced by past and present. Hermeneutics adds an interpretive element to the experience using text or symbolic form. It takes something that is already an interpretation of the experience and uses it to deepen and enrich the meaning of that which is being revealed (van Manen, 1997).

Gadamer and Heidegger considered hermeneutics so much a part of the lifeworld that it is universal; it is "the whole in which we live as historical beings" (Weinsheimer, 1985, p. 158) or a "being-in-the-world" (Heidegger, 1927/1962) where human existence cannot be considered outside the context of the world. Gadamer (1960/1975) believed reflection was the hallmark of hermeneutics. He saw reflection as staying open to alternatives and possibilities that are reflected through the hermeneutic conversation, the dialogue of thought and meaning that goes between text or experience and the one who is interpreting. When the interpreter and the text or experience are in conversation, there is a reflection of the meaning of what is. The interpreter comes to an understanding of something new. In hermeneutic conversation, that something new is being (Gadamer). Being is how the lifeworld is manifested, and we come to understand it through interpretation (Dahlberg, Drew, & Nyström, 2001). So, then, a meaningful interpretation is a reflection of being that is now understood.

The Structure of Hermeneutic Phenomenology

van Manen (1997) describes hermeneutic phenomenology as a methodology that puts language to everyday experience. It is systematically uncovering, describing, and interpreting the meaning of daily existence. He proposes six research activities that are in interaction with each other and make up the structure of hermeneutic phenomenology: (a) deeply questioning a phenomenon, (b) turning "to the things themselves" (Heidegger, 1927/1962, p. 50) to see how the phenomenon is being fully experienced, (c) finding the essence of the experience through deep and persistent reflection, (d) putting words to the experience so that it shows itself, (e) staying attuned to the question and phenomenon without being drawn away by personal experience or reflection, and (f) moving between the parts of the experience and the whole of it, so one fits with the other.

A phenomenologist begins by deeply questioning a phenomenon, asking about the essential nature and meaning of an experience.

> Inquiry is a cognizant seeking of an entity both with regard to the fact that is and with regard to its Being as it is. …Furthermore, in what is asked about there lies also that which is to be found out by the asking [das Erfragte]; this is what is really intended. (Heidegger, 1927/1962, p. 24)

The purpose of hermeneutic phenomenology is to "come into conversation with the text" (Gadamer, 1960/1975, p. 349), to be open to different questions and different interpretations of meaning.

Phenomenology questions the way we experience the world and explores the meaning of that experience. It strips away that which is not essential and leaves the fundamental meaning of the experience. For me, the purpose of phenomenological research is to study the events of every day life, and to find the significance in these events to the people with whom I work. I want, and I must understand, the meaning daily life events hold to them to be able to help them meet their unique needs. My phenomenological research question for this study delves into the experiences of birth mothers of children receiving an FASD diagnosis for their children so that, in understanding them, I can influence how the mothers are viewed by others and how others shape their responses to the experience of these women versus their own personal perceptions.

Turning "to the things themselves" (Heidegger, 1927/1962, p. 50) to see how the phenomenon is being fully experienced. According to Merleau-Ponty (1945/1962), the lived body is the starting point from which people grasp their lifeworld. It is the taken-for-granted place where people exist and from which they attend and act on the world. Merleau-Ponty felt that it's through phenomena that we come to understand this lived world. By returning to the world of actual experience, we come to understand the experience as " a process of integration in which the text of the external world is not so much copied, as composed" (p. 9). Phenomena are given meaning and significance that are shaped by context, history, other experiences, and perceptions.

To turn to the things themselves, I needed to gather descriptions by mothers of their experiences, being careful that I gathered lived experience that had not been filtered by reflection or self-analysis. A birth mother is a birth mother, whether the mother of a child with FASD, a child with Down Syndrome, or a typically developing child. Mothers share the experience of wanting to protect their children; they want happiness and success for their children. They perceive themselves as good or bad based on how their children grow and develop. They blame themselves when their children struggle, no matter what the struggle—it's what mothers do! But is there something a little more intense or somehow different in the shared experiences of birth mothers of children with FASD? And what is the significance of these experiences to the mothers? And how should the meanings of these experiences influence my work?

The mothers' descriptions of their experiences needed to be unbiased by their own preconceived assumptions of how they should have lived the experience, or by how they expect others think they should have lived their experience. The experience of the mothers needed to be presented to me as it was sensed in the moment, not as it was reflected upon and colored by expectations. The mothers needed to be able to give a clear, precise, and detailed description of their experience, so the phenomenon came to exist for me (Giorgi, 1997). The text, then, needs to relive the experience and be able to awaken recognition of similar experiences in self and others (van Manen, 1997).

Finding the essence of the experience through deep and persistent reflection. To fully understand the meaning of an experience involves reflection. "The act of understanding presents itself as reflection on an unreflective experience. Reflection is not absolutely transparent for itself, it is always given to itself in an experience" (Merleau-Ponty, 1945/1962, p. 42). When we are in the natural attitude, we place meaning on experiences, and we may not be fully aware of those meanings. It is through reflection that we challenge our preconceived ideas and are able to set aside the pre-understanding to find the essence of the experience (Gadamer, trans. 1976). Pre-reflective descriptions of an experience bring forth the hidden essence—the pure self—of an experience so that it can then be reflected upon, interpreted, and described in all its richness, yet with the knowledge that no description can fully reveal the complexity of the experience (van Manen, 1997).

In my search for the essence of the experience for the women in my study, I first needed to become aware of my prejudices and preconceptions. I needed a time of self-reflection and bracketing to understand my own related experiences. By understanding my own history—my own experiences—and the associated meanings, I was able to set aside my personal assumptions. Phenomenological reduction allowed me to move beyond my natural attitude and bring attention to the themes or constituents of the phenomenon. This, in turn, helped me to remain open to the women's experience and later to the text of that experience.

Putting words to the experience so that it shows itself. Linguistic transformation is the creative, hermeneutic process of putting words to our interpretations and insights (van Manen, 1997). Phenomenological research is embodied in written form.

> Understanding is effected and enlarged by the text; now we can see further that the text is continuously effected, brought about, and realized by understanding. The history of understanding is the effectuating history of the text. Understanding makes history, makes the past by belonging to it, and adding itself to it. (Weinsheimer, 1985, pp. 14-15)

Written text allows the reader to experience the phenomenon pre-reflectively as offered by the participants. It also allows the reader to share in the interpretation of the essence of that experience and find some level of connection and empathy with those who have described the phenomenon (van Manen, 1997). Giorgi (1997) says that "to describe means to give linguistic expression to the object of any given act precisely as it appears within the act" (p. 241).

"Phenomenology attempts to systematically develop a certain narrative that explicates themes while remaining true to the universal quality or essence of a certain type of experience" (van Manen, 1997, p. 97). We use language to put words to the experience. Language opens lifeworlds to others. Language—discourse—expands and facilitates shared understanding, and it is the way phenomena come to be known. The intent is to come to a common belief about the experience between the person doing the experiencing and the interpreter. The interpreter can then bring that belief to a larger audience. The intent is also to understand the meaning of the experience to the person experiencing it and how that meaning came to be (Weinsheimer, 1985).

Through my writing, I wanted to reveal the essence of the experiences of birth mothers to others, specifically health care and education professionals, so that they can better feel and understand the mothers' experience, and act and react differently to the mothers themselves. I also wished to help the mothers come to understand their own experience and how the essence of that experience was shared not just with other mothers receiving the FASD diagnosis for their children, but more broadly, mothers of children with other diagnoses, and even mothers in general. It may be that the birth mothers of children diagnosed with FASD could come to know a different meaning of their experience when the essence of the experience is revealed through dialogue.

Staying attuned to the question and phenomenon without being drawn away by personal experience or reflection (i.e. maintaining a strong and oriented relation) (van

Manen, 1997). A phenomenologist must stay focused to the question she has asked and true to the methodology. She must be self-reflective and able to set aside personal preconceptions and assumptions to permit the experiences of her participants to be revealed as they are lived. And she must ground both the question and the interpretations in sound theory. van Manen states that "to be oriented as researchers or theorists means that we do not separate theory from life, the public from the private" (p. 151). Gadamer (1960/1975) believed that there cannot be understanding without interpretation, or full understanding without application.

My reflections and interpretations must contribute somehow to my work and my life and the work and lives of those with whom I am interacting. To do so, my interpretations must be strong in the way they answer my research question; they must be rich in their descriptions of meaning; and they must provide a deep understanding of the phenomenon. They must be grounded in the theories of my profession and contribute to the body of knowledge of which I am a part. I must be able to apply my understanding of the meaning to the mothers of receiving the FASD diagnosis so that it makes a difference in the lives of the mothers. More broadly, I must be able to apply the meaning in my work as an occupational therapist and as a family and community health care educator.

Moving between the parts of the experience and the whole of it, so one fits with the other. "When something no longer takes the form of just letting something be seen, but is always harking back to something else to which it points, so that it lets something be seen as something, it thus acquires a synthesis-structure, and with this it takes over the possibility of covering up" (Heidegger, 1927/1962, p. 57), that is, we have truth. Truth is

40

bringing together the whole with the parts, a process referred to by Gadamer (1960/1975) as the hermeneutic circle. (See also Kvale, 1996.)

> Understanding is always a movement in such a circle, for which reason the repeated return from the whole to the parts and vice versa is essential. In addition, this circle continually expands itself in that the concept of the whole is relative and the inclusion in ever larger contexts alters the understanding of single parts. (Gadamer, p. 167)

The hermeneutic circle, then, allows revision of the truth of the whole of the experience because we can grasp a deeper understanding and integration of the parts until the true meaning is found. The ultimate goal of phenomenological research is to continuously measure the overall meaning of the whole against the meaning and significance of the parts (van Manen, 1997).

Each iteration of the event, each remembrance, must be understood in itself, but also against the whole of the experience. We move between the part, which is the present, to the whole, which is history and tradition, to come to new understanding (Dahlberg, Drew, & Nyström, 2001). Because contexts and experiences change, we can never fully understand the meaning. According to Dahlberg, Drew, and Nyström, "the challenge for lifeworld researchers is to be so sensitive to both the whole and the parts of the data and to the meanings of the phenomenon, and to write so clearly and articulately, that the inherent ambiguity of the lifework and its meaning is captured" (p. 186).

As I worked with the text given to me by my participants, I needed to be aware that my interpretations were projecting meaning influenced by the other texts I had been reading as well as my own preconceptions, however carefully I had bracketed them. It was vital to bring each interpretation of a part back to the meaning of the whole to make sure it was true to the rest of what was being revealed.

Research Methods

Participants. The interview participants were birth mothers of children who had been diagnosed with a Fetal Alcohol Spectrum Disorder. Following procedures approved by the University of Minnesota Institutional Review Board (IRB Code: 0610P94486), participants were identified via the Minnesota Organization on Fetal Alcohol Syndrome's (MOFAS) Family Seminar Series: Project Seeds of Success (Project SOS). The coordinator of Project SOS was provided with letters requesting participation. She added her statement of support and mailed the letters to potential participants.

Women who were willing to be interviewed contacted me to set up an interview appointment. During this contact, they were asked to identify a place where they felt most comfortable sharing their embodied experience. It also had to be a quiet place for recording. Prior to the interview, each mother was taken through the consent process and offered a brief explanation about my interest in the experiences of birth mothers (refer to Appendix A for the consent form). They were also told about the purpose of the tape recorders and reminded of how the transcripts from the interview would be used.

According to Polkinghorne (1989), participants in a phenomenological study are chosen because they have a deep and intimate experience with the phenomenon of interest, and they are able to reflect upon and fully articulate that experience. My interview participants were all birth mothers who had experienced receiving the FASD diagnosis for their child. However, when analyzing the interviews, one of the difficulties

I encountered was an interview done with a woman who was not yet in recovery from her alcoholism. I believe she may have been using alcohol at the time of the interview; at least she appeared to be cognitively impaired by her recent active alcohol use. Even though her descriptions were similar in content to the other mothers, if more exaggerated and intense, that interview was taken out of the analysis because the participant wasn't able to meet Polkinghorne's criteria of being able to give a sensitive description of her experience.

Study participants are also chosen to represent different populations and contexts to assure that the description of the essential structures of the experience won't change if the person or context changed. For this study, I obtained and transcribed 10 interviews, ultimately using 9. Each interview was one to two hours in length. The interviewed women included two upper middle class women, five of middle and lower socioeconomic status, and two women on public assistance. Six were Caucasian, one was African American, and two were Native American. Educationally, one had a tenth grade education, two had graduation equivalency degrees (GED), three had a high school diploma, one had some college, one had earned a bachelor's degree, and one held a master's degree. Five of the women had their children living with them at the time of the interview (representing nine children with FASD). One woman had given up both of her children, one to foster placement and one to adoption. Another had given up two of her four children diagnosed with FASD to foster care. The grown child of one woman was in the Army, and the son of another was in prison. One of the women who retained custody of her son was scheduled for court in the coming weeks and was at risk for termination of her parental rights. The time between diagnosis and interview ranged from less than a week to six years. At the time of diagnosis, of the 15 children represented in the study, 1 was diagnosed as a newborn, 5 as pre-schoolers, 5 in their elementary school years, 2 in their early teens, and 2 were diagnosed at ages 17 and 18.

Data collection. "The point of phenomenological research is to 'borrow' other people's experiences and their reflections on their experiences in order to better be able to come to an understanding of the deeper meaning or significance of an aspect of human experience in the context of the whole of human experience" (van Manen, 1997, p. 62). A phenomenologist needs naïve reports of an experience as it appears in a person's consciousness, free of the biases of the phenomenological researcher.

A researcher may choose to gather examples of the lived experience through written text, interviews, observation, artifacts (e.g. art, structures), or pre-existing descriptions (e.g. literature, journals). I chose to use interviewing for this study because I felt interviewing would allow me to mine for anecdotes that revealed deeper meaning. I could repeat or rephrase questions and take my participants more fully into their experiences in a way that couldn't happen with observation or by using preexisting written text.

Gadamer (trans. 1976) suggests that questioning increases one's openness to experiences. The phenomenologist knows that she does not know, and with an open question she seeks to reveal the many possibilities of the unknown. During the interview, each mother was asked to describe her experience of coming to know about her child's diagnosis of FASD. Interviews were unstructured. The two main questions (which were repeated when we were ready for a description of another event) were: (a) Think about when you found out that your child has FASD. What was that like for you? (b) Tell me about getting the FASD diagnosis for your child.

According to Gadamer (1960/1975), "The art of questioning is the art of being able to ask further questions, that is, it is also the art of thought. It is called dialectic because it is the art of carrying on a real conversation" (p. 331). Probing questions and requests for illuminating incidents were used to move deeper into each mother's experiences. Examples of follow up questions were: Can you tell me more about that? Can you give me an example of that? What happened next? What did you feel? What was that like? I anticipated the mothers would naturally drift into talking about their child's behaviors or the different ways their lives have changed after the diagnosis. They were redirected to the original questions about the meaning and experience of first coming to learn about the FASD diagnosis for their child.

I was mindful of each mother's emotional state, anticipating that this sharing could be difficult and painful. Women were informed that they were free to participate or not participate in the study. They were also informed that they needed to only disclose what they are comfortable sharing, and that they could discontinue the interview at any time. As a health care professional, even though I didn't anticipate anything adverse would occur, I provided a list of resources that offer support for the mothers, including community agencies such as the Minnesota Organization on Fetal Alcohol Syndrome and the American Indian Women's Resource Center. During my interviews, I did not detect cues of distress, and none of the participants asked to stop the interview. I also did not

need to bring the interview to a close early to protect the participant.

In addition to the interviews, preexisting written descriptions (poetry, video,

stories, and personal accounts) were used in a hermeneutic response to more fully

examine the themes drawn from the interviews. These items were obtained through

newsletters that contain columns written by mothers of children with FASD (e.g., *F.A.S.*

Times), autobiographies, and a video produced by the Center for Substance Abuse

Prevention (DHHS, 2004b). A book, *Cheers! Here's to the Baby* by Linda Belle LaFever,

contained a written account from a birth mother and was also used to support themes.

Reduction and bracketing. In hermeneutic phenomenology, there is recognition

that as the researcher I cannot fully separate myself from the texts that are being

examined and described. Dalhlberg, Drew, and Nyström (2001) and van Manen (1997)

wrote of the need for self-reflection to come to understand one's natural attitude toward a

phenomenon, then bracketing those beliefs so as to allow the participants' lived meaning

to be revealed. Because of my personal experience working with birth mothers, I took

time to do this self-reflection. I wrote a personal account and completed a bracketing

interview as part of the study. This helped me come to understand my own thoughts and

feelings about the FASD diagnosis as a mother, as a mother who drank while pregnant,

and as an occupational therapist and family and community educator working in the field

of FASD diagnosis and intervention. Extra care could then be taken to set aside my

preconceived notions so the lived experiences of the birth mothers I interviewed could

come through without my biases attached. Bracketing allowed me to examine the phenomenon without bringing in my preconceived notions. I became aware of my biases and personal background, and I tried to set them aside so that I could describe the phenomenon as it was experienced by the mothers without risking describing the phenomenon of receiving the FASD diagnosis as I assumed it to be.

Text analysis. Each interview was transcribed verbatim prior to theme analysis. This gave me written text to work with as I began to unravel the interviews to find the essence or essential structure of the experience birth mothers have of receiving an FASD diagnosis for their child.

van Manen's (1997) holistic examination was used for a first analysis of transcriptions in order to get an impression of the overall meaning of the experience. This was done with the precaution that I needed to remain open to the meaning of the text without imposing myself into it. The more intimately I knew what the mothers were saying, as I read the whole of the texts, the less likely I became to imposing my own meaning and prejudice to their experiences.

To communicate meaning to others, van Manen (1997) organizes the pre-reflective lived meaning shared by study participants into themes, or what he refers to as "the experiential structures that make up the experience" (p. 79). Themes are meant to simplify and capture the experience. Each theme in and of itself does not reflect the entire phenomenon but illuminates parts of the whole. To find the themes, I examined the text for words or phrases that seemed to expose the experience, an act van Manen refers to as using the selective or highlighting approach. These phrases were left in the words of my study participants and recorded beside the text so I could return to them as I tried out different interpretations of the meaning of the phenomenon. (See Appendix B for examples of text with interpretations.) I was slow to add my descriptions or interpretations because I wanted to stay open to possible meanings.

Once I had examined the text and highlighted phrases, I began to work with them, transforming them into my own words using the language of my disciplines of occupational therapy, public health, and family and community education. I then experimented with different interpretations, an exercise van Manen (1997) refers to as linguistic transformations. My attempts to re-describe the experience served to move forward the interpretive or hermeneutic process of theme analysis. Throughout this process of text transformation, I attempted to maintain a stance of openness and questioning. I also attempted to stay in a reductionist stance to avoid placing my assumptions onto the meaning of the text. I frequently referred to the narrative I'd written, and the interview I had completed, to make sure I was hearing the voices of the women and not my own voice. Moving between the whole and the parts also helped me stay in a reductionist stance.

Imaginative variation allows the researcher to change or remove what she deems as essential to the phenomenon to see if by doing so there were changes to the fundamental meaning or essence of the phenomenon (Giorgi, 1997; van Manen, 1997). As themes began to emerge, I used imaginative variation to remove or change them to see if, by making these changes, the phenomenon changed. I wanted to determine if the themes that had been described were essential or incidental to the phenomenon (van Manen, 1997). I would then try to fit my identified themes back into the texts of my subjects' interviews. This part-whole-part process of moving from theme to texts to theme (the hermeneutic circle) was used to seek deeper meaning and bring answers to my research question.

When I felt that I had abstracted all the themes and variations from the text and the meanings didn't contradict, a point that Kvale (1996) terms reaching a "good Gestalt" (p. 48), I began to look at the themes as a mother who drank while pregnant, as a family and community educator, and as an occupational therapy clinician working with this population. This helped me to see if there were missing ideas.

Heidegger (1962) and Gadamer (1960/1975) believed interpretation was essential. The job of the phenomenologist is to "construct the possible interpretation of the nature of a certain human experience" (van Manen, 1997, 41). Kvale (1996) encourages the phenomenologist to "involve innovation and creativity" (p. 50) in interpretation of text to "[enrich] the understanding by bringing forth new differentiations and interrelations in the text, extending its meaning" (p. 50). So too, van Manen (1997) suggests using what he calls experiential material to increase insight into the phenomenon of interest, allowing others to identify with and better understand the meaning of the discovered themes. As I worked with the revealed themes, I brought the preexisting written materials I had gathered to enrich and deepen the meaning of those themes.

Specifically, I brought in written materials to more deeply examine the meaning of the themes in two ways. First, I wanted to deepen the meaning of the theme itself by bringing in the voices of other mothers of children with disabilities. Then, I wanted to better understand how unique the experience of receiving a diagnosis was to women of

49

children labeled with FASD specifically, compared to women whose child has a diagnosis and has a diagnosis in which she is implicated as a cause. There is the voice of the mother, and there is the voice of the mother who caused her child's disability.

As part of my interpretation, I used etymology to trace words back as far as possible in their own language and to their earliest source to see how meaning developed. According to van Manen (1997), finding the origins of a word can often reveal the early lived experiences associated with that word. These early meanings lend richness to the interpretation of the phenomenon that is being studied. In addition to etymology, sources on mothering in general and mothering children with disabilities, including literary and visual arts, were used to amplify and deepen my understanding of my participants' lived experiences as well as transfer and apply the themes more broadly.

Giorgi (1997) warned against trying to force all the data into a single theme, but to recognize that variations can exist in the data. He felt that the "ultimate outcome of phenomenological scientific analysis is not just the 'essential structure' but rather the structure in relation to the varied manifestations of an essential identity" (p. 249). Five themes revealed themselves through text analysis, yet there were also nuances to those themes that I deemed important to understanding the full meaning of the mothers' experience. They weren't completely enveloped within the themes themselves, but they were needed to add to the richness of understanding and were included as subthemes.

Validity

During this research study, I was cognizant of several issues related to its validity. First and foremost, to increase the validity of my research, I needed to adhere closely to the phenomenological and hermeneutic philosophical perspectives. These included being mindful of the principle of openness, showing consideration for history and tradition and the biases and prejudices that may result, preventing pre-understanding from interfering with understanding, and searching for a deeper understanding of the phenomenon as it is (patiently letting the phenomenon reveal itself) by using the whole-part-whole scientific attitude of interpretation.

Openness is a criterion of objectivity in phenomenological research. "Openness is the mark of a true willingness to listen, see, and understand" (Dahlberg, Drew, & Nyström, 2001, p. 97). According to Dahlberg, Drew, and Nyström, to be considered valid research, the researcher must understand how her personal character and approach impacts how the phenomenon presents itself. Openness to the research question requires careful use of methodology and use of the literature.

Openness to oneself is an awareness of how the self can affect the research by the ability to remain focused and attentive to what the phenomenon is saying. It is the ability to set aside preconceived ideas (reduction and bracketing) and to stay attentive to the research situation. The first time this self-awareness is needed is during data collection. I needed to continually return to the question and not allow myself to be distracted into asking leading questions or questions based on preconceived ideas.

In addition, I took a great deal of care to be thorough in data collection by making sure my participants were credible and that they were able to deeply reflect on and articulate their experience without self-analysis and self-interpretation. Validity was also increased because of the type of open-ended questions I asked in the interviews and the way I conducted the interviews so as not to lead or direct responses but to listen carefully and actively.

The second time openness is required is during data analysis, when I needed to make sure I was allowing the experiences to speak for themselves (Dahlberg, Drew, & Nyström, 2001). Giorgi (1997) emphasizes that the phenomenologist is to be "present to what is given precisely as it is given" (p. 237). I needed to continually be aware of how my analysis, transformation of the data, and use of imaginative variation were a reflection of the women's experiences. I had to take care to not impose my own set of meanings onto the text.

Intersubjective openness was also a consideration. This means that I am aware that I understand the phenomenon and the research situation more than my participants, but I was able to move beyond the natural attitude that I hold, embrace a scientific attitude, and let the participants and their experiences come to be (Dahlberg, Drew, & Nyström, 2001). Again, I was conscious of the need to remain open both when gathering and when interpreting text. I was careful with the questions that I asked, and the methods I used so that they were not leading. I was also careful in casual conversation before and after the interviews so I didn't present myself in a manner that would give participants an impression that would impact their sharing. During text and theme analysis, I needed to make sure I was transforming the women's words into "phenomenological, informed psychological expressions" (Polkinghorne, 1989, p. 57), and that my themes accurately reflected the meaning of the experience to the birth mothers. In other words, I needed to make sure my methodology made sense and resulted in themes that others can accept as a valid experience of my participants.

Finally, van Manen (1997) wrote of the importance of connecting theory to life and believed application was needed for a full understanding of the phenomenon. As part of the data analysis, I needed to make sure I was being true to my discipline. I needed to transform the mothers' experiences into a language that would make the information applicable to health care and education.

Goals and Significance of Research

It is my experience that much time is spent in diagnostic team meetings on first labeling and then describing to the caregivers what the diagnosis of FASD means for their child, but there is little if any time spent in helping caregivers—mothers— understand what the diagnosis means for them. Further, an examination of the literature finds hundreds of articles on how to diagnose FASD, the impact of alcohol on brain neurophysiology, early intervention strategies, long-term outcomes, and primary prevention of alcohol use with mothers. Yet, there is no literature found in refereed journals about the experiences of mothers when the diagnosis is given to their child. If we can deeply understand and appreciate the lived experiences of mothers of children diagnosed with FASD, we can better anticipate the kinds of supports they might need and the approaches from the diagnostic team that might be most useful to them at the time of diagnosis. We can appreciate and be more sensitive that we present information in a way that mothers can hear and use. We can inform social action and public policy through an understanding of her perspectives. And we can help mothers come to terms with their own experiences and empower them to hold their experiences as valuable and meaningful.

Chapter Four: Pre-understanding and Assumptions

I remember getting called out of class where I was teaching mental health content to take a call from the school where my son was. He'd told some kids he was feeling suicidal, and then didn't show up at school. The social worker called me— she had some worried kids in her office. I remember the moment of getting the news. I remember feeling like I'd been slugged in the stomach…hot-cold, breath being taken away. Do I cry? What do I do? I couldn't even think of a plan. I was immobilized; stuck. I couldn't figure it out. Do I go home? Stay? Who do I call? Do I immediately go out to the school and see if they are doing it right? How dare I do that? How can I because I've already screwed up as a parent. Why else would he be suicidal. Who do I tell? Who do I get support from? Do I tell family? God, no! Do I call my husband? He'd just be upset and no help. Do I tell colleagues? That I'm a bad mom? They'll know I'm not what I said I was, that I can't do my job because I can't even see when my own kid needs help. What a horrible mom I am – a horrible person. (personal reflection on getting a label for a child; bracketing interview)

Pre-understanding

"When we think of the world, it is always the world already containing us thinking it" (Cogan, 2006, p. 5). We cannot completely take ourselves out of the natural attitude; we cannot completely bracket all of our pre-understandings because we are human and of the world. The best we can do is to increase our self-awareness of how we investigate and describe a phenomenon to reduce our biases both in the questioning of the phenomenon and in the analysis of the text (Dahlberg, Drew, & Nyström, 2001).

Whenever we begin to examine a text or try to find meaning in an experience, we already have a formed idea—a prejudice—of what that meaning is. These subjective feelings and preferences may cause us to come to premature or incomplete understanding of an experience, preventing us from really understanding how it is lived through. Further, Gadamer (1960/1975) suggests that we "project a meaning of the whole as soon as the initial meaning is indicated" (p. 236). In other words, prejudices cause us to anticipate meaning. We change our anticipated meaning when faced with text that doesn't fit with what we expected or makes no sense given our initial understood meaning. Until the essence of the thing we are examining is revealed to us, our idea of its meaning freely changes as we examine it.

This is where the hermeneutics of hermeneutic phenomenology begins. Understanding of a phenomenon starts with becoming aware of the pre-understandings that we bring with us. We cannot completely free ourselves from the natural world; nor would we necessarily want to. But we do want to question it, to see how it might be influencing deeper understanding and ultimately influencing how we use that meaning in our daily lives and work. These insights and understandings can then be set aside to allow an examination of the essence or universal meaning of the phenomenon that has now been revealed. The essence is what makes the phenomenon under study unique and different from other phenomena (van Manen, 2002). And we want to make sure we are uncovering the essence of the experience and not reflecting our own past experiences and unrecognized prejudices and beliefs.

It is in that context that I completed a bracketing interview conducted by a colleague who was also studying phenomenology. Some of the questions that were asked in my bracketing interview included: (a) Tell me about a time when you were faced with a potentially bad diagnostic finding; (b) Tell me about when you were pregnant. What was that like for you? (c) What are your impressions of a good pregnant mom? (d) Is there such a thing as a good drinking mom?

During transcription of this interview, I was surprised at the intensity of some of my opinions about mothering and mothers' behaviors during pregnancy. I was not critical in the sense of condemning mothers' behaviors, but I was, possibly, too open and forgiving of those behaviors. Another surprise was the extent to which I depersonalized my own behaviors as a mother, as a mother who drank during pregnancy, and as a mother receiving a label (suicidal) for my son. It was extremely difficult to get down to my pre-reflective experiences. But once there, the pain of those experiences seemed as fresh as when they happened well over a decade ago. Knowing this, then, about myself helped me anticipate how I might color the meanings of what I heard from the women I interviewed.

Assumptions Associated with This Study

I found that as I thought about this study, I was also carrying some specific assumptions that went beyond my pre-understanding of the phenomenon itself. I needed to also analyze these assumptions, and then make sure they didn't influence how I was reflecting on the text and uncovering the themes.

Methodological assumptions. I made the assumption that the mothers who were the study participants wanted to make meaning out of their lived experience of receiving a diagnosis of FASD for their children. Part of making that meaning would be to share. I assumed mothers would be willing to talk or write about their experiences, making a phenomenological approach possible (van Manen, 1997). I assumed that the birth mothers would have a shared lived experience and that they would be willing to give me the gift of telling me about it, that they would be able to articulate that experience, and that they would share honestly. I also assumed that I would be able to establish enough trust with the women to have them feel sufficiently comfortable with me to share their deepest experiences and the associated meanings.

Madison (1988) speaks of rational judgments that can be supported by persuasive arguments. I assumed the texts I chose would be representative of the experiences of birth mothers and would hang together as arguments supporting the themes I defined and described. I assumed that I would be able to reconcile any themes that seemed to fall away from the developing picture of the mothers' lived experience and that I could develop a coherent and accurate interpretation of those experiences that would inform current practice and future research efforts (Madison).

The most significant assumption I made was that hermeneutic phenomenology is the most appropriate and reasonable research methodology to answer my research question of exploring the lived experience of birth mothers receiving the FASD diagnosis for their child. I believed that I could only come to a deep understanding of their experiences through their pre-reflective sharing, interpreted through a hermeneutic response.

Topical assumptions. I assumed that deeply understanding this lived experience would be useful in meeting the needs of birth mothers, and that diagnostic teams would find the information useful and important enough to rethink their post-diagnosis processing meetings. Typically, once a diagnosis is made by the team, a conference with the parents is scheduled. The results of the assessment are shared by the team, and planning begins for the management of the many medical, social, and school problems of these very complex children. While this child-focused process is set up for the good of the child and the pragmatic needs of the health care team, the protocols dominate the needs of the mother. She is likely having a strong emotional response to the meaning of the diagnosis. She may not be hearing what is being said. Her feelings and needs are frequently disregarded. To be more effective, we need to create a diagnostic process that is more mindful of her unique needs, fears, concerns, and challenges.

The FASD label is one that is heard over and over each time the child doesn't meet a developmental milestone and each time the child struggles to do what is right. I assumed that if trainers, health care professionals, and educational specialists were aware of who each of their clients might be and how each might be experiencing her child's diagnosis, we would be more cognizant of the language that we use, what our words might trigger emotionally for each mother, and how much time and space she needs to be able to hear and process what the label means to her and to her child. Only then can she begin to move forward to help her child. We need to ask ourselves when and how we should be providing information. Where is the mother emotionally? How much time does she need before she gets to a place where she can hear what to do for her child? What language will reach her? What does she need for resources?

I assumed that each mother also could benefit from understanding the mothering experience for others like her. She might come to realize that she is not unique in her shame and sadness. This understanding could help to normalize her feelings and thoughts, and it could change her self-perception of being bad and without redemption.

Having reduced and bracketed my pre-understanding of what it is like to be a birth mother receiving a diagnosis of FASD for her child, I was ready to examine the texts of the mothers.

Chapter Five: Articulating the Themes

Flutterings

Slight of movement
minute flutterings
flicker over my stomach;
as imagination takes
on passing butterfly's wings.
It's the beginning of one very new.
An early germinal stage,
the foundations of something
so much bigger to come....
Rudimentary hiccups
of one so slight.
Invisible behind my bump grows,
an immature being -
I've seen it
at scan stage.
Underdeveloped,
a miracle -
all manmade.
My future,
my hopes,
my dreams.
My child.

(Anaisnais, n.d.)

A child is conceived and a woman is transformed instantly to a mother. Whether planned and longed for, or unplanned and seen as a burden, each unborn child holds a promise for the future, and each mother wants her child to fulfill that promise. But mothers are not always successful. Because of misinformation held by themselves or given by others, because of addictions or lack of adequate coping strategies or errors of judgment, or because their pregnancy was unanticipated and mothers didn't know they were pregnant until too late, a child may be born with FASD and will struggle in every day life.

This study explored the meanings mothers hold for the outcomes of their behaviors during pregnancy. Specifically, it explores the meaning of receiving the diagnosis of FASD for their child—a diagnosis made possible solely because the mother did something during her pregnancy that damaged her child. Revealed through the interviews of these mothers of children with FASD are the essential meanings of this experience of receiving the FASD diagnosis. In a search for these meanings, I needed to interview mothers, transcribe those interviews, then live for a while with the written text, reading and re-reading until the meanings became evident to me.

Five specific themes emerged from the analysis of the transcripts. For the women, receiving a diagnosis of FASD for their child is a process, not a point in time. The process begins before the diagnosis is given. The first theme, *something doesn't seem right with my child*, describes the sense of dread that something is wrong with the child. Then the words are spoken, and the consequential meaning of the diagnosis shifts from child to mother (in the theme *I can't believe this is happening to me*) and back to child (with the theme *I can't believe I've done this to my child*). The theme *I need you to see me, hear me, help me* reflects the experience of the mother with the health care provider who made the diagnosis. The moment of hearing is replayed each time a new problem emerges or another milestone is missed. To the mother, the receiving of the diagnosis is a lifelong process, reflected in the final theme *I can't fix it; I can't make it better*.

In the remainder of this chapter, I will explore the five themes as they were revealed to me. All of the themes were nuanced. I have attempted to fully describe the nuances of each theme while avoiding attributing multiple meanings to a single theme.

Something Doesn't Seem Right with My Child

For the mothers in my study, their experience with receiving the FASD diagnosis often came before the words were actually spoken by a health care professional. It started as an inkling that their child was not measuring up to other children. The perception of wrongness, sensed somewhere in the mothers' body and spirit, because of things seen or perceived in their child led to questions and to a search for answers. Merleau-Ponty (1945/1962) believed that "ambiguous perceptions alone emerge as explicit acts: perceptions, that is, to which we ourselves find a significance through the attitude which we take up, or which answer questions which we put to ourselves" (p. 281). Often there were no clear indicators that the child had this problem or that disorder; for many mothers, FASD was an unknown condition. But theirs was the perception that something was wrong and they needed to take action. A study participant said that she didn't "know how I knew, I just knew; like a connection of mother intuition." Others spoke directly about knowing and searching for answers:

> So when the PT [physical therapy] wasn't working, the OT [occupational therapy] wasn't working, the speech wasn't working...he's now in sixth grade with a second grade reading level. So, you know, he kept going backward so they put him in LD [classroom for students with learning disabilities]. And that really wasn't doing anything but frustrating him, because they were trying to get him to do grade level's work, and he couldn't do it. I used to call him a very slow processing computer. And I said, "We need to do an assessment on him."

> I kinda knew something in my heart was, something's not right with him, and so I kept asking questions, how do I find out what the alcohol did to him?

There were also times when a friend would make a comment about possible FASD, or the mother would have attended a presentation and come to the realization that this could be the reason for her child's struggles. One mother found out about FASD from a friend who was a foster parent. Comparing notes on their children, she came to the conclusion that this was what she was facing with her oldest son. Another found out about FASD while seeking her own treatment for chemical dependency:

> Once he was born and I got myself into treatment, the things that they said could happen to a child from a mother drinking and on drugs, I started thinking then. I started, oh really praying and hoping that it didn't damage my child, but here in Minnesota, he started having these behaviors. People coming in asking, "Well, what's wrong?"

As with any mother who senses there is something wrong with her child, these women went in search of answers in spite of knowing that the possible answer would implicate them as the cause. Marit said she "was terrified. When I started asking for help, I thought I would be crucified. I was so shameful" (DHHS, 2004b). Yet the need to get the diagnosis overshadowed that fear. Julie "needed to be sure; I needed to know what to do. I couldn't live with the guilt of knowing something was wrong and not doing anything about it" (DHHS).

As the participants in my study shared with me, I wondered if what they experienced was similar to the experiences of mothers of children with other disabilities. Did all the mothers have a sense that something was wrong, or were they told there was a problem? Did they pursue this sense or was help thrust upon them? What would make them come to the point where they felt it imperative to have their children evaluated for a possible disability?

I remember my mother telling me something didn't quite look right with my toddler son's eyes. One was remarkably bigger than the other, and was I sure there wasn't something wrong with him mentally? Her comment drove straight to my heart. I had been secretly thinking that maybe he was cognitively delayed, but I hadn't dared say the words out loud for fear that they just might come true. I had been searching for clues that he was somehow not right, but at the same time searching for signs that everything was fine. Now the words were out there in the air, and it meant I had to face the fact that something didn't seem quite right with him. I had to take some sort of action to find out what was wrong, even as I feared what the answer might be. It ultimately turned out to be nothing, and he's actually intellectually gifted, but I still acutely remember the moment of her question and the clutching fear in my heart.

In an effort to more deeply understand the theme *something doesn't seem right with my child*, I searched the literature for resources describing the experiences of mothers receiving a diagnosis for their child for conditions for which they could be seen as culpable. What came to mind were HIV/AIDS, genetic conditions such as hemophilia and Fragile X, and thalidomide. I was unable to locate first-person accounts by mothers, although I did find a few articles discussing mothers' attitudes gathered through semi-structured interviews and surveys. The richest accounts of experiences came from mothers whose children were diagnosed with conditions that were once considered the result of poor parenting (autism, cognitive disabilities, and learning disabilities) and mothers of children who had physical disabilities or chronic illnesses.

In *A Difference in the Family: Life with a Disabled Child,* Featherstone (1980) draws on interviews and autobiographies to explore parents' journeys toward understanding their new lives with children with disabilities. In a way similar to my personal experience, the parents about whom Featherstone writes begin their journey with the fear that there must be something wrong with their child.

> Hoping to reassure themselves, parents collect facts and observations that buttress their hopes. At the same time they watch warily for symptoms, for surer indications that something is wrong. Karen Junker, whose third child, Boel, seemed subtly different from her older brother and sister, describes her efforts to settle her nagging doubts. Unable to formulate her suspicions, she observed Boel constantly—"spying" she called it, remembering the covert, anxious intensity with which she watched her daughter, even in sleep. "It was a sort of sly hunt for symptoms, of what I didn't know.' (p. 14)

The sense of apprehension that something is wrong seems universal to mothers of children who are found to have hidden or unexpected disabilities. Three mothers of children with three different diagnoses (autism, cognitive disabilities, and a learning disability) shared their angst in personal accounts of their struggles to come to terms with identifying their child's disability:

> Something, I sense it acutely, is wrong. There is an absence of things. Small lights burning out. The creep of an indecipherable dimness....I supposed that mother's intuition was a hard, certain thing, a perpetually replenishing reservoir of basic instinct. If there were problems, the gut would howl it. If there were risks, the heart would rattle. I remember thinking I was suddenly much too tall and much too thin to be a mother, and that no amount of stooping could bring me into my son's space. (Kephart, 1999, p. 51)

> I think I was the last to perceive that something was wrong. She was my first child and I had no close comparison to make with others. She was three years old when I first began to wonder....I can remember my growing uneasiness about my child. She looked so well, her cheeks pink, her hair straight and blond, her eyes the clear blue of health. Why then did speech delay! I remember asking friends about their children, and voicing my new anxiety about my child. (Buck, 1950, p. 13)

> The recommendation for a full neurophysiological evaluation doesn't really surprise me. There are numerous signs of David's difficulties I've done my best to ignore, frantically overlooking what should have been obvious. Where David was concerned, I spoke only to people who would reassure me. (Weinstein, 2003, p. 117)

These mothers searched for signs of deviance, excused delays, and grabbed onto any indications that their child was normal. Unlike me, their relief came not in finding out their child was normal, but in the relief that there was an answer and the anxiety of not knowing had passed. Their fears had been validated, and they were no longer powerless because of the unknown.

What is it like as a mother to have your concerns validated? It's one thing to have a sense that something is wrong with your child and to actively seek and get a diagnosis. There is a sense of being listened to and somehow respected for your mother knowledge. It's quite another to know there is something wrong but to be disregarded or to struggle to be heard.

Many of the women in my study spoke of not being heard when they reached out for help with their child's behaviors.

> I was constantly trying to reach out and look for support, to look for answers to my questions, to look for help, look for ways of handling different situations because of his behavior and I was always getting stopped. It was like me being totally blind and reaching out there and not finding nothing. So when I got the diagnosis, what a relief. Now they can give me some of those answers and get the truth.

Another mother had a sense that her son was struggling with more than the usual teenage angst and went in search of answers. For her, the process of getting someone to listen to her was more difficult than actually getting the diagnosis.

> The emotional front end work is the hardest part of the whole process. For me it was. Acknowledging. Telling other people. And then getting put off because of that. Ignored because of that. And then having that sense of knowing inside, "No, I really do think this is part of it." As a woman I rely on intuition and a knowing kind of a sense. And when other people just ignore that, it's—abusive isn't the

right word, but it's like this rejection. It's rejection of who you are when you're taking that risk to come forward with the information.

Several poignant narratives in *From the Heart* (Marsh, 1995) spoke of the pain mothers had of knowing something was wrong with their child and being ignored, having concerns discounted, or being blamed for being a poor parent. The following examples taken from the book express the mothers' distress: "Being heard is the single most important idea. Every time I had a conflict it was about being heard, in varying degrees. Jeremy had cancer and no one would listen to me saying the kid was sick. I went here, I went there, we took him to the hospital, we were told, 'There's nothing to worry about'" (p. 3). "It's being believed, just that. That is the essence of it for me. That it's really like this, and I'm not just making it up" (p. 6). "The professional's line of questioning was pointed. I felt that he had already decided that Asher was emotionally disturbed as a result of my poor parenting. I cried for days" (p. 30).

While actually receiving a diagnosis was a painful event, to be finally heard brought relief. The mothers in my study now had validation for their mother intuition, had permission to grieve, and could move forward with a sense of direction and purpose to dealing with their child's problems.

> It's like there's an answer, you know? Maybe it wasn't because I was a bad parent the whole time and because I wasn't…I mean I'm an educated person and I did everything I could when I was raising him to learn about what I thought was going on with him and advocate for him in the school system, and advocate for him with the doctor and to get the proper mediation and all. When I got the diagnosis, it's like, "Well maybe I did the best I could with the knowledge that I had, and now I have to look at it differently. The damage is done whatever the damage is and now I can just help him to move forward in life."

Pearl Buck (1950), in her autobiography *The Child Who Never Grew*, writes, "the first cry from my heart when I knew she would never be anything but a child, was the age old cry that we all make before inevitable sorrow: 'Why must this happen to me?' To this there could be no answer and there never was" (p. 6). It is this pain that is at the heart of the second theme of the mothers' experience.

The mothers with whom I spoke first heard the label of FASD as it applied to them personally, even as they came to understand the ramifications of the disorder for their child. What will others think about *me*? What have *I* done? How will *I* go on? What did *I* do to deserve this thing that is happening to *me*? One mother said, "I put myself to bed for a week. Beating myself up." In the video *Recovering Hope* (DHHS, 2004b), Kathy shared that, "my whole world shattered. It was like a tidal wave came over me. I went into a panic mode." Another mother in my study called it "the most devastating moment of my life. Cuz I did that to him. I did that to my son. I wanted to die." Still another recalled going to a meeting to find out more about FASD and what it meant for her son, but she was caught up in what it meant to her.

> Most of the time I'm sitting there thinking what a lousy mother I am to have done all of this to my child. And I'm fighting back the tears. And still trying to listen. And I'm thinking, OK. I'll take my time and read [the information]. But then it makes me feel so—like I—I'll use the term unfit mother. That gets in the way. That's one of the reasons why I haven't sat down and tried to read it. Because all that keeps going through my head is you're a lousy mom to do this to your kid, and there's nothing you can do about it.

Theirs was the sense of being alone with the diagnosis. Many mothers felt that they had been handed something unbelievably painful, then left to deal with it alone.

I remember breaking down and crying. Some lady came up and hugged me, and she comforted me and she said it's gonna be alright. And to this day I don't know who that woman was, but it was something I needed cuz I was there all alone. All I wanted them to do was tell me how I could help him survive.

What is it that mothers experience when they first hear the words Fetal Alcohol Spectrum Disorder applied to their child? Many of the women felt the pain of hearing the diagnosis both physically and emotionally. Merleau-Ponty (1945/1962) described the body as the place where one "brings into existence...takes upon herself, space, object or instrument" (p. 154). According to him, the lived body is the starting point from which people grasp their lifeworld and are able to attend and act on that world. The experience is in the body and that bodily experience is shaped by context, history, other experiences, and perceptions. The mothers with whom I spoke had an immediate visceral reaction to hearing the words of the diagnosis:

> It was like taking a physical hit and then nothing else, everything else kind of goes. It's all fuzzy in your head. You don't have clear impressions. It's like going into shock. They're talking, but it's just bouncing back and you're kind of in your head going, "Oh my God, oh my God, what have I done? What have I done?"

> It hits you like a brick wall the day you find out. Or like one of them round balls, wrecker balls...the opposite of exploding. It's like I wanted to sit down and be depressed and "God, what do the doctors think of me?" They were both looking at me, four eyes on me and I'm going, "I bet they think I'm a terrible mom."

Theirs was the gut-wrenching physicality of emotional pain that defines the experience. Something bad has happened that has shaken their self-image of mother, their context of what it is to be a mother, and their perceptions of how they will now be viewed in their mother role.

Again I wondered, is this experience unique to FASD? I looked to the literature for the experiences of mothers who took thalidomide while pregnant. I assumed that the

70

mother's experiences with the outcome of prenatal thalidomide use would be closer to that of mothers who drank prenatally than to those mothers of children with other pregnancy or birth-related diagnoses. Thalidamide was a medication used in the late 1950s as a sedative and to reduce the nausea of early pregnancy. It was later found to be a teratogen. Roskies (1972) completed a several years' long phenomenological study of mothers who had taken thalidomide. Similar to alcohol, some of the mothers knew there was potential for fetal damage; most did not. The mothers' reactions were similar—the immediate physical and emotional pain, the attempts to deny and blame, and the sense of being in it all alone.

To more deeply explore the possible uniqueness of the birth mothers' experience with receiving the FASD diagnosis, I looked to the literature on other child diagnoses where mothers have been implicated in the etiology of the condition. The literature on HIV/AIDS consistently point out that the distress mothers feel, at least in the first year of their child's life, has more to do with their own feelings of stigma and their own physical health, than with what the diagnosis means to their child (Miles, Burchinal, Holditch-Davis, Wasilewski, & Christian, 1997). The HIV status labels the mothers for what they might have done to develop the infection, including drug abuse, prostitution, or sexual promiscuity. Such stigma results in the mothers spending less time caring for their children and more time and energy covering their HIV status (Bunting, 1996; Dougherty, et al.,1990; Ostrom, Serovich, Lim, & Mason, 2006). One mother summarized her child's (and her) HIV diagnosis, stating, "you can never be normal again. You have to fight for that. People will label you. I haven't changed, but the labels will change you. You can't change how everyone else feels" (Ingram & Hutchinson, 1998, p. 95).

Genetic conditions, especially those that are X-linked rather than recessive-gene linked, elicit self-blame and the focus of the mother on the stigma of being a carrier (James, Hadley, Holtzman, & Winkelstein, 2006). The self-blame, fear of stigma, and attempts to conceal the disease exemplify a mother's initial reaction of the search for meaning for herself when she first hears her child's diagnosis.

I also looked at narratives of mothers whose child received other lifelong diagnoses. Each mother spoke of the unbelievable pain she experienced at hearing the words, "Your child has this diagnosis, and *you* must learn to live with it."

> I can't come in from the dismal rain with my hair all wet and my nerves shot and my son in my arms, yet miles away. And I can't say things are good and I can't say things are bad, and then blame it on myself when no one, maybe, is to blame. I can't say those things. I can't even speak. I can't believe how deep the hurt goes, or how black things look, how broken. (9, 1998, p. 63)

> I remember walking the endless hall again alone with the child. I cannot describe my feelings. Anyone who has been through such moments will know, and those who have not cannot know, whatever words I might use. Perhaps the best way to put it is that I felt as though I were bleeding inwardly and desperately. (Buck, 1950, p. 23).

> There is the problem of one's own self misery. All of the brightness of life is gone, all the pride of parenthood. There is more than pride gone, there is an actual sense of one's life being cut off in the child. The stream of generations is stopped. (Buck, 1950, p. 27)

> My professional expertise offers me no solace or special understanding. How can I be a doctor and have a child with so many problems? I did all the right things, I studied hard, I didn't try to hurt anyone. (Weinstein, 2003, p. 13)

> Like Picasso's *Weeping Woman*, I feel my face breaking up into its component parts, learning a new topography of pain. (Weinstein, 2003, p. 15)

As the mothers in my study struggled to reconcile the FASD diagnosis given to their child with their own behaviors and responsibility for their child's disabilities, they also agonized over their perceptions of how others might see them. Merleau-Ponty 1945/1962) wrote that "perception goes straight to the thing and bypasses the colour" (p. 305). The mothers no longer perceived themselves as just mothers. Their colour—those qualities and characteristics that make them unique as mothers and women—no longer carried value. They now perceived themselves as bad and expected that others labeled them bad as well.

> People are thinking I'm a bad mom just like I did when I first found out. I always feel like I have to explain myself and try to make them think that I'm not a bad mom that I know is running through their heads—I feel like it's running through their heads.

> God, what do they think of me? What are those doctors thinking of me, like looking down their noses at me, or they think I'm the most terrible, terrible person.

> I wasn't one of these people. I didn't sit in the bar every night of the week and just get totaled. The guilt is unreal. But it was the first time I had to acknowledge to others that there was that level of consequence to my drinking.

> [My sister] hasn't a clue. And if she does, she still makes it the way she talks to me—I get the sense that she blames me. That I'm not such a good person, much less a good mother.

It's not just my fault. The theme, I can't believe this is happening to me, is played out as the mother sinks into the pain, grief, and regret she is feeling for what might have been her life and what she must now face with her child with a newly diagnosed, life-long disability. Her life as she knew it is over and she must make new meanings and new realities for herself. A sub-theme, it's not just my fault, is embodied in both denial and looking for ways to pass the blame.

Kristie Alley plays the role of Sally Goodman, the mother of a child with autism in the film *David's Mother* (Randall, 1994). At one point in the film, she lashes out at her sister for pushing her to accept that she is not at fault for her child's disability, and that she deserves to have a life apart from her child. She demands that her sister explain how she could be so positive there is no fault.

> They don't have a clue what caused David to be born with scrambled eggs for brains, but *you* know it wasn't my fault. I wish I knew that. I wish I knew it was the fluoride in the water, or the asbestos in the ceiling, or the lead in the paint. I wish I knew it was the joint I smoked when I was carrying him, or the wine I drank that I was so sure wasn't going to hurt him. Or that I have some screw up in my genetics, in my chromosomes. Then I'd know who was at fault.

She is looking for someone to blame, suggesting that maybe there are two Gods, "one that cooked his brains and one that kept him that way." Her anguish at her son's disability is palpable. Even as Sally Goodman struggles with her son's disability and tries to find a cause to blame, she (and we) know there is little evidence pointing to any specific cause of autism. How much more must be the pain of the mother who actually knows she caused her child's disabilities?

In the video *Recovering Hope* (DHHS, 2004b), Marie expressed a common myth about FASD, saying, "deep down in my bone marrow, I thought how can a well-educated, well-brought up woman possibly have a child with Fetal Alcohol Syndrome?" One of the mothers in this study separated herself from the diagnosis of FASD when she explained that:

> [Now that I have the diagnosis] I don't have to deal with it anymore. I don't have to deal with ignorant professionals. [I don't have to deal with them] regarding my own use and its impact on my son. I can define it at any point if I want to. I'd say I feel relieved that I—like this little chapter is behind me, and now I can move forward.

Another mother acknowledged her alcoholism but denied the extent to which it controlled her life and affected her children. She fell back to rationalizing her use of alcohol and attempted to draw a boundary between the bad—the no-good alcoholic—and the good—I was too young to know any better.

> In my mind, I would go back to when I was pregnant with him, and I didn't handle it well. I just…it's that whole younger person cuz with alcoholism you don't mature as quickly as you should, and it was still kind of a holdover from that teenager. I'm invincible. This can't happen to me. I wasn't one of *those* people [her emphasis].

Two other mothers also described being powerless against their own addictions, in essence blaming the addiction for the outcome of their pregnancies. One mother explained that "both my pregnancies weren't planned. And I tried to quit drinking once I knew I was pregnant. Myself, personally, I have…a problem." The other said she "didn't know about fetal alcohol, but I knew about drugs. They could damage the baby. I did know that. But I was just, was in a state of mind that I didn't know how to deal with my problems back then."

Most of the women interviewed wanted to make it clear that their child having FASD wasn't just their fault. They implicated their doctors for giving bad advice. One woman "got the message from my doctor that it was okay to drink a little bit each day. One drink at the wrong time. I'd quit drinking just before a buzz. I didn't think he was going to end up this way." She went on to say that she was angry at "the doctor telling me not to worry about it and me breaking a child." Two other women felt they had unfinished business with their doctors.

75

One of the steps I will take at some point is to call the family practice doctor that gave me really, really bad advice 18 years ago. So he doesn't—if he's continuing to give bad advice, he needs to know that it's a mistake. That'll be a closure piece for me.

I wanted to strangle the doctors. Cuz when I found out I was pregnant, I was in the process of a divorce, so of course I was hitting the bottle. So when I found out I was pregnant, I said "Do I have to worry about Fetal Alcohol?" "Oh no, you'll be fine." So we have a child that has OT, speech, PT starting at the age of one. And the behaviors got worse and worse.

I can't believe it's what they say it is. Most of the women wrestled with applying the diagnosis of FASD to their own child. They talked about having a diagnosis but still not being sure that's what they were coping with. They felt confused about the diagnostic criteria and how the criteria applied. They struggled to see how the diagnosis fit with their particular child. And they expressed a disbelief that they had drunk enough or at the right time to cause FASD. One mother requested an assessment, fully thinking her son would not fit the diagnostic criteria because "of his somewhat limited exposure." Another doubted the diagnosis as well:

> I just think of my lifestyle and how that just doesn't match up, you know? So people drank all through pregnancy, smoked all through pregnancy. When I found out I was pregnant I stopped all that, and just was careful though my entire pregnancy to eat right and not drink. I honestly think that prior to knowing I was pregnant, I probably had something to drink maybe once or twice. It just doesn't add up.

I Can't Believe I've Done This to My Child

It wasn't that many years ago that mothers expected to lose some or all of their children to illness and injury. In our modern world, we expect that our children will be born normal and healthy; it would be more accurate to say we expect our children to be born perfect. If that doesn't happen mothers look for blame—in themselves for having done something wrong during pregnancy, at their families for overlooking something they should have insisted be corrected, or at their doctors for something done, not done, said, or left unsaid.

Dally (1982) describes motherliness as warmth and sensitivity toward the child. To be motherly—a good mother—is to protect, enhance, facilitate success, and to give of one's self for the betterment of the child. A bad mother is self-serving and destructive toward her developing child.

The good mother-bad mother dichotomy is found in the third theme that emerged from the interview text. In this theme, the mothers agonized over decisions they made during pregnancy that ultimately damaged their child. They struggled with their inability to protect their child and their sense of being blamed and judged by others just as they blame and judge themselves.

> Something like FAS; somebody is gonna come back and say it's your fault. It doesn't matter what kind of mother I am now. I did this and it's my fault. Doesn't matter if it was one night before I knew I was pregnant. It's my fault. It's acceptable for a man to be drunk. But a woman? Especially a mother? It's a reflection of how people consider them as a mother. You've done something unforgiveable. There's no excuses. There's no vindication. There's no cure. You made this mess and you can't clean it up.

> I beat myself up. And now that he knows, there's sometimes he says, "you did this to me," which makes me feel about this big every time. If I knew I was pregnant I wouldn't a drank. But I did. I feel about this big.

> I look at them and I cry because of what I did. Just crying about shame, guilt, hurt, wondering. I'm supposed to protect them, take care of them. How could I hurt them? How could I damage them? How could I destroy them? How could I ever take care of them?

This feeling is not unique to mothers of children diagnosed with FASD. Kathy, in

From the Heart, wrote:

When my son was diagnosed with autism/pervasive developmental delay (PDD), I anguished over my possible role in this disability: Was it something I ate when I was pregnant? Was it that severe allergy I suffered in my seventh month? Is it genetic, did he inherit it from me? Was it the protracted labor and C-section delivery? Or was I merely a woefully inadequate mother? (Marsh, 1995, p. 56)

Mother is one of the universals of mankind. We all have experienced a mother; we have personal knowledge of a mother and a sense of what a mother should be. Saying the word mother conjures up images of both good and bad mothers. The Virgin Mary, even though unmarried and pregnant with Jesus, is depicted as the model of serene and perfect pregnancy and motherhood. The ancient mother goddesses were believed to be filled with love, compassion, and mercy. In her phenomenological study on mothering across the lifecourse, Francis-Connolly (2004) asked her participant mothers to define the perfect mother. Words such as "god-like" and "incredibly encouraging" reflect the level of unattainable and unrealistic images that are associated with the ideal, perfect mother.

As the mother of three, a grandmother, an aunt, a health professional who has worked with at-risk pregnant women and new mothers, and a friend to many mothers, I have felt and have heard the stories about being labeled a bad mother. We live in a world where there is little hesitation in identifying where we all fall on the good-bad mother continuum. Mothering and motherhood have been idealized, and in that idealization, there is permission from others to judge the behaviors of women. The protruding stomach of a pregnant woman brings not just the pats on the belly (even by total strangers), but advice on how to be a good pregnant woman. So too, the baby in arms or stroller seems to give permission to others to judge a mother's competency. Mothers also do it to themselves.

"Sooner or later the child disappoints you, perhaps even terrifies you with a small sign of distorted development or a subtle betrayal of temperamental weakness" (Lazarre, 1976, p. 181). In her book *The Mother Knot,* Lazarre wrote of her uncertainty about her adequacy as a mother, and as a mother of a child who might not be perfect. She wrote of her fear that if her child is not perfect, somehow neither is she. Featherstone (1980) writes that the "whole culture supports a mother in the opinion that her children are what she has made them" (p. 71). Mothers credit themselves for their beautiful and successful children—and are full of guilt over the child who is not. And public opinion supports this.

Many parents—mothers as well as fathers—live their lives again through their children. It's easy to see this at soccer and hockey matches and during recitals and performances. Parents want their children to be winners, to be the best or brightest. They will then have proof that they did a good job parenting their child. The temper tantrum in the grocery store, the failed grade in school, or the missed basket at a critical moment in a basketball game are all a reflection of the failure of the parent to provide enough of whatever is needed to create a winning child. As mothers, we want the proof that we are good mothers. Most often we get the message that we are at fault for something bad that is seen in the child. It's not the child, it's the mother. With FASD, the finger of blame points squarely at mothers.

> I brought him into this world but at the same time I kind of ruined his chances was how it felt because the doctor was like, you know, this is the normal curve, and this is probably what he's going to do. It just kind of felt hopeless.

> Before we had the diagnosis it was because I'm a bad parent because I'm not disciplining him right or whatever. Then when I found out this diagnosis I just

79

feel horrible. Because of something I did he's going to have to live with this for the rest of his life and it's going to challenge him and it's going to make life difficult and it's going to impact everything he does for the rest of his life.

Just knowing that I'm the cause of this for my child, for my son, makes me feel very inadequate....It's hard to explain; I just feel like...I'm sorry about it. But that doesn't seem to be enough. There seems to be something more I should be able to do.

In her work on mothering across the lifecourse, Francis-Connolly (2004) spoke of the angst mothers in her study experience when they don't say or do the right things with their child. She found that the women in her study were constantly comparing themselves to an ideal mother. The ideal mother is described by Dr. Benjamin Spock and other baby experts as ever-present, inexhaustibly patient, all providing, and acutely sensitive and responsive to her child's needs (Francis-Connolly, Marshall, 1991). Falling short of this level of perfection, her study participants expressed a feeling of guilt. Birth mothers of children with FASD are unable to even get to the point of being guilty for a lack of perfection—they did not do the right things for their child even before birth.

Although dated and psychoanalytical in flavor, the book *Inventing Motherhood* (Dally, 1982) reflects the thinking that is still evident in present day. Mother is to blame. Dally devotes several pages of her book to explaining how devious, depressed, anxious, or restricted and restricting mothers create children who are neurotic, withdrawn, under-socialized, and mentally ill. Even though this line of thinking is no longer followed in modern day psychology, we as mothers have not rid ourselves of this belief. Nor has society, for the most part, found a more satisfying explanation for why some children seem to go bad. There needs to be an explanation, or all of our children are vulnerable. It's better to blame the mother for the child's behavior than to consider our own child at risk for such behaviors. Lazarre (1976) wrote in *The Mother Knot* of the impossible task of being a good mother.

> There is only one image in this culture of the "good mother." At her worst, this mother image is a tyrannical goddess of stupefying love and murderous masochism whom none of us can or should hope to emulate. But even at her best, she is only one limited sort of person, not the vast treasure house of human possibility which would be the stuff of a creative and nourishing cultural myth. She is quietly strong, selflessly giving, undemanding, unambitious; she is receptive and intelligent in only a moderate, concrete way; she is of even temperament, almost always in control of her emotions. She loves her children completely and unambivalently. Most of us are not like her. (pp. xxi-xxii)

Living with guilt and shame. As mothers, we strive to be seen as good. What then, of the mother who has caused damage to her child? She certainly cannot be considered a good mother. I believe that all mothers experience some level of guilt and blame. We take on the guilt whenever we perceive that our child doesn't meet the expectations set by ourselves or our society. Merleau-Ponty (1945/1962) wrote that "perceptual experiences hang together. The perception of the world is simply the expansion of my field of presences" (p. 304) and that "appearance is, within me, reality" (p. 377). In the context of his words, if I feel guilt and shame, I will perceive that others are blaming me. I feel guilt and shame; that becomes my reality and I will internalize it, whether or not the perceptions are accurate. And I will believe the world supports that self-perception. "Our body and our perception always summon us to take as the centre of the world that environment with which they present us. But this environment is not necessarily that of our own life" (Merleau-Ponty, pp. 285-286).

Heffner (1978) wrote about the "universal guilt of mothering" (p. 26) that comes from the mother's fear of being unable to adequately meet the needs of her dependent child, and that this inadequacy will cause lasting harm to the child. Whenever a mother sees problems with her child, she immediately assumes it's her fault. There must have been something amiss in her body, or something she did or didn't do in managing her pregnancy. There is the added guilt and blame that comes with being the parent of a child with disabilities. She and those around her wonder—in silence or out loud—what she did to cause the damage. With FASD, the disabilities are her fault; she in fact did do something harmful to her baby. What must it be like to be the cause of the disability? Three of the mothers in my study described their guilty feelings, saying:

> Underneath was that kind of river of just the rethinking. You just kind of go to the mind flashes at nights, you know, when I was really early in my pregnancy that I was like, nothing's gonna happen. That I was drinking and my behavior wasn't responsible in terms of an up and coming parent, so you just kind of flash back to that, and it just kind of ate at me underneath.

> I put [the diagnosis] on the back burner, and then something brings it to the front burner, and it simmers a little bit again. Instead of something past tense, it makes it present tense. It's raw. Raw is simmering. Maybe being more in touch with the emotions, like they resurrect themselves. So feelings that I have of remorse, or feelings that I have of…I think the feelings that are the hardest are seeing your own kid suffer.

> I love my babies so much, and there's been a lot of times in the past where I look at them and I cry because of what I did; what I chose to do.

When a diagnosis of FASD is received, the ability to mother is called into question, both by others and by the mother herself. After all, she has done something bad to somebody else—her own child. Most of the interviewed mothers spoke of the shame they experienced. One mother "wanted to go hide in a corner and never come out. Never, never. I mean it was one of those things where I figured that he was better off without me, cuz all I ever am doing was screwing up." Another acknowledged that "if I could go back and change things, of course I would. And the thing that really bugs me is that I knew there was a possibility of damage. It's like the last thing I need is another child that I really don't know how to take care of."

Guilt, defined by the *Oxford English Dictionary* (2006), is knowingly committing an offense or sin. In Judges 13:7, the Bible admonishes against drinking because of the damage that will be inflicted upon the child. "Behold, thou shalt conceive and bear a son, and now drink no wine or strong drink." So too, the Talmud (200-500AD) advises that "one who drinks intoxicating liquor will have ungainly children." Advertisements in restaurant bathrooms, metro bus stops, and billboards warn mothers not to drink when pregnant. A child with FASD is an outward sign that the mother has damaged her own child with her behaviors—she is guilty. She is, or can be, judged. One mother "tries not to [tell people her sons have fetal alcohol syndrome] but when you've got a 12-year-old following you screaming at the top of his lungs, crying in the middle of the grocery store, and they're like 'Do you need some help?', 'Is he OK?', 'Now why's he crying?'" "He's 12 and he's got Fetal Alcohol Syndrome. This is the only explanation." Another has a "sense of—remorse—or guilt around that. Because, you know, because he struggles so much around that. And what part I played in it."

Guilt is about what you did, but shame is about who you are. It is being wicked, disgraceful, dishonorable, and without reputation (*Oxford English Dictionary*, 2006). One mother expressed this shame when relating what her sister said to her.

> My sister told me, "Jesus Christ, [name], get off the bottle. Do something." And I tried and tried. But I couldn't. And the more I tried, the more I couldn't. And you know, to be honest with you, when I took that drink—all I would do is cry. I was

hoping I would maybe have a miscarriage. That I wouldn't have had this happen. But these kids have to be born.

Guilt comes through the message that a mother must think first and foremost about her child's needs, with those needs being most important. If those needs are not met, the mother is responsible for causing irreparable harm. There is a right—good—way and a wrong—bad— way to meet a child's needs, and mothers cause damage when they do it the wrong way (Heffner, 1978).

Do other mothers with children with disabilities experience the same guilt? Mothers whose children have HIV/AIDS, hemophilia, or other genetic conditions relate feeling a sense of guilt over the transmission of the disorder. They feel stigmatized and blamed. There is often also an added element of blame by others; fathers blame mothers for X-linked genetic diseases (Banis, Suurmeijer, & van Peer, 1999; James, et al., 2006; Madden, Terrizzi, & Friedman, 1982), and society blames mothers with HIV/AIDS for the perception held that these women have lifestyles that contributed to their infections (Ingram & Hutchinson, 1998; Mayers, Naples, & Nilsen, 2005; Miles et al, 1997). As with prenatal alcohol use, the amount of guilt and stigma experienced by the mother seems related to whether she lacked knowledge of the impact of her behaviors or felt her behaviors were due to poor character (Miles, et al.).

I feel judged by others for what I've done. According to Merleau-Ponty (1945/1962), "the other person's thoughts are certainly his; they are not of my making, though I do grasp them the moment they come into being, or even anticipate them" (p. 354). The guilt and shame often causes the mother to feel judged, wondering and anticipating what others must think of her. Mothers of children with disabilities bear the scrutiny of both family and the public, especially if the impairment is obvious to others. They often face disadvantage by virtue of their role as mother. They are the ones who typically seek a diagnosis; follow through with intervention plans; and explain, re-explain, and explain again the history of the disability. Mothers are judged by the nature of the disability, and by their ability to provide perfect mothering in spite of that disability. Mothers are often seen as the root cause of many disabilities; in the case of FASD, they are the cause. FASD is completely preventable, so the child's behaviors are directly linked to the mother's behaviors and actions. One mother stated that,

> Regardless of what anyone says, I love my child. I may not be able to show it the way I should, I suppose. But I love my child. I love my boy. It's part of my unfitness as a mother. I don't know how to try to—I know my sister tells me I can never make up or try to compensate, and help my child in every way that I can to—overcome it.

She also felt judged by others in a FASD parent support group. "I felt like I wanted to just disappear, to dissolve when they broke it [FASD] down for us. Cuz most of the other parents that were there were foster parents, or they had adopted a child that had been diagnosed with FAS or FAE."

The *Oxford English Dictionary* (2006) defines judgment as deciding what is right and what is wrong—what is good and what is bad. To be judged is to be criticized by others, often with the other assuming superiority. Judgment is associated with punishment. You have done something wrong; you must be punished. The mothers in my study, to a one, spoke of feeling judged by others.

> These people are thinking I'm a bad mom just like I did when I first found out. I try to make them think I'm not a bad mom that I know is running through their heads. Or I feel is running through their heads.

It doesn't matter what kind of a mother I am now. I did this and it's all my fault. Doesn't matter if it was one night before I knew I was pregnant. It's my fault. I think a stigma exists. It's a reflection on how people consider me as a mother. You've done something unforgiveable. There's no excuses, no vindication, there's no cure. You made this mess and you can't clean it up.

I don't know if I cried for sadness or for my shame of what I did to him. Where can I go now? God, what do they think of me, what are those doctors thinking of me, like looking down their noses at me, or they think I'm the most terrible, terrible person.

I now understand what I'm dealing with. Merleau-Ponty (1945/1962) wrote that "prior to and independently of other people, the thing achieves that miracle of expression; an inner reality which reveals itself externally, a significance which descends into the world and begins its existence there, and which can be fully understood only when the eyes seek it in its own location" (p. 320). Mothers in my study came to understand that the diagnosis was real and wasn't going to go away, and they began to accept what it meant for their child.

Most of the mothers, while still dealing with a sense of their own badness, were also able to talk about moving forward with their lives. They spoke of self-forgiveness through understanding, relief in knowing a diagnosis so they could help their children, and a desire to share their knowledge with others in an effort to reduce other mothers' pain. One of the interviewed mothers acknowledged her culpability, yet moved quickly to a self-forgiveness that came with understanding the FASD diagnosis.

I wouldn't say I dealt with shame. I don't feel shame. I feel honest. I feel forthright. I can forgive myself. I have forgiven myself. I was ignorant about what I was doing. So I don't have to deal with that stuff. If he dies, if he, well if he does, depending on what happens in his life, if he eventually becomes—if he quits using and gets his life together, then that'll be easier for me. So his success is wrapped up in how I feel. And he isn't very successful right now.

Another mother, interviewed in the video *Recovering Hope* (DHHS, 2004b), used the diagnosis to move beyond the shame and guilt and to use it positively. Kathy admitted that "once correctly identified, it changed our whole world. We had spent 16 years talking about what she can't do. We're not going to do that any more." Another mother in the video explained why she needed to overcome her guilt and shame. Penny felt the "need to be totally honest. By being honest, I get the correct information, and then I can do something [to make a difference in my child's life]".

A mother in this study was pragmatic about her son's diagnosis, and although still self-blaming, was able to dismiss others' judgments. "I don't care what they think. I got it down on black and white and these are the experts. They can help me. I can put them in my back pocket. Then later on I can use them to help me cuz now I have to help [my son]."

Many of the mothers had been searching for a long time for answers to their child's behaviors and difficulties and felt a sense of relief in the knowing. On getting the diagnosis, one mother felt that "now that it's in place, they can tell me how to help him." Another was relieved that:

> There's an answer, you know? Maybe it wasn't because I was a bad parent the whole time and because I wasn't… I mean I'm an educated person and I did everything I could when I was raising him and learn about what I thought was going on with him, and advocate for him, and get the proper medication, and all that. Maybe I did the best I could with the knowledge I had.

In spite of their shame and guilt and the fear of being judged, the mothers in my study were willing to set aside their own pain and figure out how they could be the best mother possible for their child with FASD.

Many of the women wanted to share their new knowledge with others, even as they risked being blamed for their child's disabilities. Theirs was the desire, almost a need, to prevent other mothers from experiencing the same pain they are experiencing, either by somehow preventing FASD or by being present for other mothers to ease their struggles. They grappled with what to do with the information they had about their child. Who should they tell and what would that person think of them? And would it change anything in the telling?

> I had to decide who I was gonna take the time to try to explain the things to because I didn't like it when people make comments about what their opinions are without the knowledge. You know, ignorant comments about things. I had to make sure I was in the right place to be able to talk to someone about it so that I wasn't defensive, and I wanted to educate people, and I wanted people around my son to understand.

The mothers felt that sharing would help them heal—help them let go of the guilt and pain so they could be better able to help their child have a productive life. One mother described having

> little secret doors all over the place of different feelings, different thoughts, and so slowly, I kind of let some of them out so that I don't have to close that door again on it. It was there, so then it seems to me like I cried and I felt it. But always when I say it I cry because that pain comes with it all the time. And then, then it's like it's made me just a little bit stronger to move forward to open up just a little bit more.

I Need You to See Me, Hear Me, Help Me

Merleau-Ponty (1945/1962) wrote that

> there is one particular cultural object which is destined to play a crucial role in the perception of other people: language. In the experience of dialogue, there is constituted between the other person and myself a common ground; my thoughts and his are interwoven into a single fabric...Our perceptions merge into each other , and we co-exist through a common world. It is only retrospectively, when I

have withdrawn from the dialogue and am recalling it that I am able to reintegrate it into my life and make of it an episode of my private history. (p. 354)

Language is a powerful tool. According to the *Oxford English Dictionary* (2006), language is the vocabulary of a discipline, a community of people speaking a common language, or words expressive of censure or disapproval. Language communicates through words, manner, and style of expression. To communicate is to share in something. There is mutual participation in the exchange of ideas, knowledge, facts, or ideas (*Oxford English Dictionary*). The women in my study, sensing that something was wrong, went in search of answers. They sought validation for their intuition. Yet when the answer was given, it was not given—communicated—in a way that was useful to and respectful of the mothers. Often this resulted in a cycle of inadequate and inappropriate communications, and a sense of not being heard, of being discounted, and of being judged.

> I've been getting stonewalled by this pediatrician. Like, I keep knocking my head against a wall and she's not gonna help.

> Just don't give me the diagnosis and send me out the door. That was the hardest thing when I found out. And not be told where you can go for help, or this is who you contact. Instead of just this is the diagnosis, this is how it's probably gonna be, and have a nice day. Now what? It was just kind of sending me out into a snow storm with no coat or anything, nothing to help me figure out what to do.

The need for respectful communication and an empathetic connection with the diagnosing health care provider was also found in several stories in *From the Heart: On Being the Mother of a Child with Special Needs* (Marsh, 1995).

> Things seemed *terrible*. My eyes and ears told me things were terrible, but no one was talking to me about it. No one said, 'This is really bad." I felt I was the only one saying it, and that I was a weak person for having done so. I began to feel crazy. (pp. 26-27)

I left the meeting totally traumatized. I had arrived there with a great concern about my son's development. The professional's line of questioning was pointed. I felt that he had already decided that Asher was emotionally disturbed as a result of my poor parenting skills. I cried for days. I withdrew from contact with Asher as much as possible. I felt crazy. (p. 30)

The women in my study spoke about wanting and needing to be heard, yet they also needed time to hear what was being said to them. Often their initial reaction was to think of themselves and sink into their own pain at knowing what they had done to their child. Their internal dialogue obliterated the words of the health care provider. What the heath care professional deemed as important information to give immediately after the diagnosis was not heard.

You get a bomb shell that then you're stuck out there waiting for the report. I don't remember what they said. What did they say I should do? What? What should I? And I still really don't remember that appointment real clearly, other than saying OK, what do I do? It's like taking a physical hit and then nothing else. Everything else kind of goes to…it's all fuzzy in your head. You don't have clear recollection. You don't have clear impressions. It's like going into shock. You just don't have that clear recollect or anything. It's just, you know, and they're talking to it, but it's just bouncing back and you're kind of in your head going, "Oh my God, oh my God, what have I done? What have I done?" So there, at that point, meaningful communication does not happen. It just doesn't.

Linda LaFever (2000) dramatically told of her experience with hearing the diagnosis of FASD for her son, and her reactions to the health care team giving the news.

I wanted to hit them all and make them hurt as badly as I did! Bound inside my prison of guilt and grief and shame, all I could do was retaliate silently in my vindictive thoughts. Today I get to add to my portfolio of maternal achievements the notable distinction of having singlehandedly and irrevocably destroyed the life potential of my youngest child! Again her words pierced my thoughts. "Linda, as a team we'd like to spend a few minutes explaining exactly what FASD is and what it means in terms of his needs and his limitations. Would that be all right with you now"? All right with me? Now? It had been less than three minutes since the world as I knew it ceased to exist. No thank you very much, it would not be all right with me. "Linda," she began, "Fetal Alcohol Syn…blah, blah, blah…"

fading, fading, fading in and out of my ability to stay focused. I only nodded in the direction of their voices.

Many of the women in this study talked about the manner in which the health care provider told them about their child's diagnosis. Merleau-Ponty (1945/1962) identified the phenomenon of "ambiguous perceptions...perceptions, that is, to which we ourselves give significance through the attitude which we take up, or which answer questions which we put to ourselves" (p. 281). Regardless of the manner of the health care provider or team, the mothers felt judged and blamed and the dialogue took on an adversarial and paternalistic flavor.

> They judge and make decisions right away about what I am and have done, and then I feel more shame and guilt and shut down and push away.

> God, what do they think of me? What are these doctors thinking of me; like looking down their nose at me, or they think I'm the terrible, terrible person. But I don't care what they think. I got it on black and white paper and these are the experts. It's not all about me anymore; it's about [my son].

This does not appear to be unique to women receiving the diagnosis of FASD for their child. Mothers who are seeking information about children with other diagnoses also gather these messages from their health care providers. Weinstein (2003), in the book *Reading David*, got the message through non-verbal communication. "Tears form and twitches escape when I say, 'It's very sad; he's very special'. Dr. Martin and his assistant Sharon nod, smiling, the way they have nodded one thousand times before to parents who cannot give up the idea that their children are unique. It is a TV smile—seemingly sincere, but empty" (p. 33).

Weinsten (2003) also expressed how different is the perception of the mother than what might be intended by the health care professional when a physician, excited by

91

finding the elusive diagnosis for her son, shared the diagnostic findings with her. *"God; what a pompous ass. Look at him. He's so pleased with himself, all puffed up with what he knows.* From the other side of the table, that mother side of the table, intellectual enthusiasm looks like cruelty" (p. 25).

"The Hippocratic oath may exhort the doctor to do good; it does not tell him how to act in a situation where the baby's needs, the mother's needs, and society's needs may have to be balanced against each other" (Roskies, 1972, p. 68). The reality of which Roskies wrote was played out for the mothers in my study. They spoke of a need for the health care provider to communicate a helping stance, to be empathetic to their situation, to assuage their guilt and fears, and to be present with them in their pain. For the most part, they did not feel this happened.

> I was there all alone and I was just like, all I wanted them to do was tell me how I could work with my child so that I could help him, help him survive. And I just remember the guy saying to me, this is the way your son is, you know. You can't change him and one day he'll probably be in prison and there's nothing you can do about it.

> It was just the way the doctor put it when we were in there. It kind of felt like from his point of view that it was just gonna be completely difficult and wasn't gonna be a very good life.

> We talked a little bit and she said, "Well, you've got the FAE and that's it and deal with it and get over it." She was like "look lady, get a grip. This is what you're dealing with and it's not gonna change."

The mothers in this study had mixed feelings about using the system to get the answers they sought. According to Heffner (1978), mothers typically want to have the opinion of specialists; however, the specialists in turn may not want to hear what she has to say. "Too often, the message given mothers is that a child with a problem by definition has a disturbed mother" (p. 134). Most of the mothers in my study had already experienced ineffective interactions with the medical, educational, or social service systems, and they felt that the systems didn't recognize or in other ways discounted their needs.

> The first time I went looking for help, [the health care provider] was kind of treating me like I was this hysterical mother. It made it really tough for me. You know, just that patronizing kind of—he didn't listen; he didn't believe me. He's just talking to me like I'm emotional. And he's like "it's not gonna go away, you know. He will turn into this and this and this and there's not gonna be any happy rainbow answer for you."

> The system can just destroy you and beat you down and then I think of those parents that don't have the education. They don't have the fortitude and the knowledge and the will to push forward and to advocate.

Even as the mothers searched for information and wanted validation for their fears, the very things they needed to share with their health care provider were the things they were reluctant to bring to the conversation. Some of the mothers feared what would happen when they expressed their concerns and disclosed their prenatal alcohol use.

> I needed to know [the diagnosing doctor] supported me and would answer my questions and wouldn't threaten me with taking my child away. I still get guarded with who I share with and what I share, especially when it comes to professionals.

> I'm not feeling like I'm coming from a place of power, but more or less a victim of the system. I don't want [my child] or myself to become a statistic or fall through the cracks in the system. I don't know what to do about it.

I Can't Fix It; I Can't Make It Better

Merleau-Ponty's (1945/1962) concept of relationality (lived human relations) is a transcendence of the self. It is how we are in relationship with others. Each birth mother moved from what the diagnosis of FASD meant for her and the shame and guilt of being a bad mother, to knowing it wasn't just and only about her. Sally Goodman, the mother in the film *David's Mother* (Randall, 1994) cries for what could have been, for what was lost because of what is. She knows her son is damaged, and she believes that what she has is as good as it will get. She wonders, as do the mothers of this study, about what the diagnosis would mean for her child for a lifetime. This sense of impotence, fear, and grief over the future was part of this final theme shared by the study participants. Theirs was the knowledge that the FASD diagnosis had become a permanent part of their lives. One of the study participants summed up the mothers' feelings when she said that, "[It's] not going to be a 24-hour thing. It's going to be like months, years maybe. I'm still dealing with it. I have to deal with it every day." Another, the mother of a nine-year-old, looked ahead and wondered,

> Okay, now what? Now how am I going to deal with this? Am I going to get this child out of my house by the time he's 18? No. Besides, it's on a piece of paper telling me he'll never live by himself. I'm not going to do this. I can't handle this. Cuz he's already gotten to the point where I'm pulling out my hair. And they're saying he's going to get worse than he is right now.

These mothers live with the wish that things could be different, but they know that they will be reminded of their child's diagnosis each time he or she tries to learn new things or faces the typical challenges of normal development.

> It never goes away. Not any day I have to go see my kid, you know? To court on Wednesday, last night I went to see him [in jail]. So no, every time you see your kid it comes back. Every time you get a phone call. Every time—and it doesn't define who he is to me. But it's a struggle. I don't know if it will ever end. It was kind of like this—when you're launching a kid, you want them to be semi-together, you know? And then you feel that, okay, my work's done, to a certain extent. I mean of course you always keep parenting, but I'm not legally responsible for this kid anymore. But when kids are in their senior year of high school, it's kind of a finality thing. And he's not going through any of those typical rites of passage. His rites of passage are treatment and jail, and lots of chemical use. That's what his rites are—so you don't really get a sense of success as a parent, like okay, job well done. It's just—I feel it's a chaotic situation that's

going to keep cycling through again and again and again. With him—doing stupid things that impact other people.

Facing the forever struggle. In *The Mother Knot,* Lazzare (1976) captures the angst of mothering a typically developing child. How much more is the anguish of parenting a child with lifelong disabilities?

> I had felt the milestones gathering behind me. I call these moments periodic and occasional. Only in retrospect do they gather together in one mass, giving the illusion of long, unified periods of time; so that women will say to you—ah? But to watch a child grow! Or frightened by your unpleasant descriptions of the early years, they will say, but when she took her first step! When he said his first word! Still, they are really only moments, as separate and occasional as the slight, suggestive snow flurries of October. (p. 157)

Children with FASD can become happy, successful, and productive adolescents and adults. However most will struggle with lifelong disabilities that interfere with their ability to become independent. Mothers of children with FASD may not experience the successes we dream of when we look at our babies and watch them grow up. The frightening future stretches ahead. One mother tells of her son's future. "You're going to be a fetal alcohol child for the rest of your life. It's all new. Everything is new." In a moment of despair, Ann Wallner (2002), the mother of a child with FASD, writes in *Another Year of Crises and Choices:*

> I'm angry. We've just made it through another year I wish I could have skipped. Again. Crisis after crisis. New depths of grief and pain. Yet again. And I wonder if it will ever be different. A recurring phrase that others offer us in puzzled tones, and that my husband and I have uttered to each other with sighs of despair, is, "It doesn't stop for us, does it?" (p. 3)

The parents who spoke in *A Difference in the Family* (Featherstone, 1980) feared the ultimate long-term outcome for their child with disabilities—institutionalization, victimization, a life dimmed by an inability to navigate the world or even complete daily living skills. While they are able to manage the day-to-day crises associated with their child's disability, the fear of the future for their child overwhelms them.

The sense that the child is facing a "forever struggle" seems to be a universal idea felt by all mothers with children with disabilities. Mothers with children diagnosed with the HIV/AIDS virus fear for their child's future without them as well as their child's life itself. Theirs is a struggle with the implications of stigmatization and discrimination that often results when they disclose as they search for services (Dougherty et al., 1990; Mayers, Naples, & Nilsen, 2005; Miles et al., 1997). Mothers of children with hemophilia also face the fear of the life-long consequences of bleeds, a fear that includes pain, the development of physical handicaps, and possible death (Banis, Suurmeijer, & van Peer, 1999; Madden, Terrizzi, & Friedman, 1982)

Three mothers of children with autism, cognitive disabilities, and a learning disability express their fears over the futures of their children.

> Tomorrow, when we wake up, nothing will be any different than it is now, at this haunted hour. And the next day, and the next day, maybe things will never change. Or maybe Jeremy will engage, emerge, evolve, and maybe I will learn how to build a household of rules, learn how to mother firmly, learn how to interfere with the precious patterns of my son's endangered world, learn, even, how to trust his growth to someone else, to therapy—where will we find it? How? No one, not even science, can edge us closer, help us see. Words, approximations, muddy crystal balls are all there is. Words are it for us right now. Everything else is the same. (Kephart, 1999, pp. 74-75)

> When the inevitable knowledge was forced upon me that my child would never be as other children are, I found myself with two problems, both, it seemed to me, intolerable. The first was the question of her future. How does one safeguard a child who may live to be physically very old and will always be helpless? (Buck, 1950, p. 24)

> Good-bye travel soccer team, good-bye Rhodes scholarship. In one minute David has gone from someone "normal" to someone who is on the treadmill of

developmental difficulty, a child whose pleasure will be bounded by the schedule of his remediation, of his need for help. (Weinstein, 2003, p. 33)

How might that be a different experience for a mother whose child will have a life time of struggles because of her? One mother knew that her son was "going to have to live with this for the rest of his life. In my rational mind I'm like, I can't do anything about the past, and I didn't do it on purpose and all of that other stuff, but you know, still…"

Another mother of a child diagnosed with FASD was already thinking ahead, even though her son was still in pre-school.

> He might not be able to drive and he might not be able to live on his own, and these are all the things you have to expect, and I was just thinking that he wasn't going to have a future as I would hope, and I knew it was going to be hard. It's going to be forever having the extra people needed and I thought back to my high school and the kids that were in the behavior class.

To mother is to watch over, protect, nurture, and sustain; it is to care for and to protect (*Oxford English Dictionary*, 2006). We can kiss a "boo-boo" and it magically goes away. We can listen to and comfort sobbing teenagers when relationships fall apart. A mother's touch brings safety and security.

The mothers in this study spoke of remorse and sadness for what they had done to their child. Their sadness was not so much around what the label of FASD means for them as a mother, but it was over the long-term impact of the diagnosis for their child, and their inability to make the reality different. One mother summed up the feelings of all the mothers when she stated,

> I think the feelings that are the hardest are seeing your own kid suffer. That's the hardest part. The hard part isn't forgiving yourself. The hard part isn't my feelings. The hard part, the painful part for me is seeing him struggle, which

makes me sad, because when you watch a person struggle with things that are easy for other people, struggling to just do daily life—it's just painful to see that. It's just, just kind of a sadness, but—you know. It's like you're powerless. Just like you're powerless. Just like I'm powerless over his addiction. So you just understand the powerlessness. When it's done like that, it's done. Some things you can go back and fix, but some things you can never go back. That's the saddest piece. That he will always have some struggles. That he can't not have. Oh, he'll mature out of some of his struggles, but—we can't fix—I can't fix him.

One somewhat surprising thread that came through the mothers' shared stories was the message that they wanted to change things for the future for other women. They had received a difficult diagnosis for their child, and wanted to spare other women that pain.

This is terrible. This is a tragedy and it still happens. The reality is there is always going to be an issue. So let's find a humane way of handling the diagnostic and then set up a process so it doesn't have to become a double tragedy.

I'm not the only one out there struggling with this issue. They can learn from me. They can learn. They can learn how to avoid these situations [related to getting a diagnosis].

I cried and I felt it, but always when I cry and the pain comes with it all the time, then it's like, it's made me just a little bit stronger to move forward to open up a little bit more. I want to go to the different reservations and speak…take a group of women and to touch the birth moms.

What Is the Experience of a Birth Mother Receiving an FASD Diagnosis for Her Child?

After interviewing the birth mothers in my study, I spent a great deal of time living with the texts of those interviews, trying out different themes and examining variations and nuances. Five themes finally emerged and held up to repeated scrutiny. *Something doesn't seem right with my child* is the mother's intuition, gleaned from subtle behaviors, comparisons with other children, and gut feelings. Once those intuitions are brought to light and labeled, she grieves for what she has lost—her perfect child and her dreams of what the future might have been. Alone in her pain, she looks for ways to escape or deny the label in the theme *I can't believe this is happening to me*. Ultimately, the mother moves into self-blame, guilt, and shame—*I can't believe I've done this to my child*. She judges herself and she feels judged by others. The theme *I need you to see me, hear me, help me* reflects the experience of the mother with the health care provider or diagnostic team that gave her child the FASD diagnosis. Finally she comes to know that *I can't fix it; I can't make it better*. She has been unable to protect her child from a lifetime of challenges.

I'd like to close this chapter by imagining what it's like to be a birth mother, living the experience of receiving the label of Fetal Alcohol Syndrome for my child.

> I'd been watching my child for a while now. He didn't seem to be like the other kids. He's got these behaviors that I can't understand. Nobody seems to want to hear me—they seem to listen but they don't hear. How can I make them understand? He's different. He looks different, he moves different. I don't quite know how to describe it, but I just knew there was something wrong. I could feel it down to the marrow of my bones. There was something wrong.

> My God, what have I done? I really didn't expect to hear what I heard. Fetal Alcohol Spectrum Disorder. I feel like those words have slammed me up against a wall. I can't think. I can't see. I can't hear what the diagnostic team is saying. It's just a fuzzy noise. I know I should listen. But I can't. Did I really drink that much when I was pregnant? What will I tell my husband? What will I tell my parents? My friends? I can't believe I drank enough to cause this. It's my doctor's fault. He said a drink a day was okay. I was just following doctor's orders. Now what am I going to do? My heart hurts. I feel the pain deep into my very center. Why do they keep talking? I can't hear; I need to think. Please be quiet and let me think. This is my child, my life you are talking about—we are people and you just changed everything with your words. How can you be so...so clinical about all of it? Can't you say a kind word? Show a little compassion? Or just be quiet!

> What will people think about me? I'm sure they'll think I'm the worst mother possible. My poor child. I've caused so much damage. He'll never be able to do well in school. Maybe he'll never be able to live alone, have a job, get married.

His whole life will be a struggle. I hurt so much for him. He'll have so many problems to deal with because of me.

So this is why my child has had so many problems. It's all my fault. This thing will affect him for the rest of his life. And there will be so many challenges that come with it. He won't be ready to hear this is what he has to deal with. He's going to hate me forever. I had so many hopes and dreams for him. All that is lost. My perfect child will never be. Now I need to figure out how I can help him be the best he can be.

Chapter Six: Summarizing and Reflecting

Withers

She withers
 just a wisp of who she was

The smile folded into solemnness
hiding feelings too painful to feel
  Feelings festering to the surface
  Scabs picked off
  Feelings slapped down
  Growth pushed back

Mom, I am but pieces
  broken
and shattered
and empty
  Lifeless.

She laughs
 with a laugh that moves even the angels

I really did it this time, didn't I?
  Even in a place of safety and maintenance
  I cannot succeed

I have fallen for their nothingness.
  Of being a less than
  no expectations - no reason to contribute
  the purpose of living you say Mom
  everyone is worthy of giving
   a thought - I am not smart
   a smile - I am not good
   an action - I am no longer able

She walks frail and medicated
  Still wanting to speak to the audience
  She has been called to give testimony to

And in slow mental processing
  fogged with medication she speaks
  of being slated for helpless
   that became hopeless
That safety brought no comfort -
  come forth to shelter
  from the storms of life.

And to my child
I whisper I love you
and I pick her up
    and swing her tiny body around
And I know in my heart
    there is very little left
And together we flee
    for miles and hours
    and hours and miles

And now she sits in a chair
    with wheels - restricted
    while she builds
        her strength
        and courage
    to allow the Master's hand
    to reform the broken pieces
    and rearrange them new

And I "with her" will help her
walk again
and stand tall again
and laugh with the laugh of angels again
and again we will march for the voiceless
and be thankful we have
    been given the privilege to see the unjust

And always a spring time will
bring new growth on old stems
Because we know our water runs deep
and our roots know their source

(Kulp, 2008)

In her poem *Withered,* the mother of a child with FASD shares with her readers

the pain her child is experiencing as that child struggles with disabilities caused by her

mother's prenatal alcohol use. The anguish of the mother is also evident. Hers is the child

damaged for a lifetime. She can try to fix it, as mothers are wont to do, but she cannot

ultimately protect her daughter from the pain and suffering that she herself, as an

expectant mother, caused.

I set out in this study to try to more deeply understand the meaning of the experience birth mothers have when they receive the diagnosis of FASD for their child. I felt that if I could somehow understand that experience, I could become a more empathetic health practitioner and family and community educator. And I felt that I could share that insight with others who work with these women, so that with deeper knowledge, my colleagues would appreciate and respect the mothers' pain. I also felt that if the mothers themselves understood they shared a common meaning in their experiences they could be gentler to themselves and to each other.

I began my study by looking at the literature on FASD. It quickly became evident that while there is a great deal of literature on the diagnosis itself—the etiology as well as how the diagnosis is made—we in the field are only at the beginning of examining what to do about it as far as preventing it in the first place or intervening once a child has been impacted. More importantly for this study, there has been no work done beyond personal narrative (blogs and editorials) that looked at the birth mother's perspective of having a child with FASD. (One article was found that used a small sample to explore the adoptive parents' experience.) There was also nothing I could locate that examined the birth mother's experience of receiving the FASD diagnosis for her child.

Because I needed to shift my thinking away from the children and the diagnosis itself, I did a short foray into the literature on women's drinking to better understand what keeps a woman doing those very behaviors she must know are damaging to herself, if not her child. I also wondered about the good mother-bad mother dichotomy. Where did it come from, and why does a woman still struggle to overcome a belief that if she is not perfect as a mother she has failed? As I began my text analysis, I also found myself wondering if the themes I was finding weren't the common experiences of any mother of a child with any disability. Do all mothers feel a personal loss and personal sorrow for their own changed lives? Do they all feel shame and guilt over the birth of a child with disabilities regardless of the cause? Do they mourn the loss of the perfect child as they reshape their lives around a child who will be forever disabled?

I chose to use phenomenology to look at the experiences of birth mothers. I wanted to find out what it meant to them as birth mothers to hear the words "your child has Fetal Alcohol Spectrum Disorder." I believed that their experiences would go beyond shame, that which appears to be the predominant way of thinking. This approach allowed me to use the words of the women to try to come to a deeper and richer understanding of the meanings the mothers hold. Phenomenology allowed me to go beyond the natural attitude so that the women's experiences could be revealed to me in all their nuances and richness. It could only be through this full understanding that I could hope to influence decision making that would impact the lives of the women with whom I spoke.

The Journey

One of my original concerns about doing this study was being able to find women willing to talk with me. Although I am known in the state for my work with FASD, and many parents know me from parent education classes, I was asking mothers to talk with me about a very personal and painful thing. I actually had many women calling in response to advertisements for volunteers. There were tears on the telephone, and beginnings of stories that had to be stopped in lieu of the need for consents and a more conducive interview arrangement.

However, there were several times where I showed up as per our agreed upon arrangements only to have the mother not appear. In some cases, the interview did not come to fruition; apparently, and I can only surmise, the mother decided not to go through with the interview. These women did not return calls, and I chose not to pursue them too ambitiously; they were clearly not ready to share their stories. In other instances, the interviews ultimately happened. The chaos that is the life of a mother, and especially the life of a mother with a child with FASD, often precludes the niceties of being able to spend time just chatting with another woman.

For me, a difficult challenge of using the phenomenological approach was the need to stay true to the words of the women—to be open to the meaning of the experience to them, without my preconceived understandings and prejudices. It was critical for me as the researcher to be self-aware. I share some common experiences and have worked in the field for many years. I naturally carry biases and pre-conceptions. These needed to be examined and set aside if I was to truly understand the women.

The nature of qualitative study doesn't permit generalizations but is an attempt to reflect the experience of the study participants, examining those experiences to uncover themes that represent the meanings of the experience. Five themes emerged for the birth mothers receiving a diagnosis of FASD for their child, beginning with the knowledge that something is not right with the child—there is something different about the child. When the cause of that difference is identified and labeled, the mother first hears what it means to her, then what it means to her child, and finally what it means for their lifetimes. Throughout the process, she is impacted by her interactions with the teller of the news. This process of hearing the diagnosis may happen in a matter of minutes, or it may happen over days or even years. And it may happen again and again as the child misses important milestones, or health care practitioners and educators repeat the words "Fetal Alcohol Spectrum Disorder."

Wanting to Be Heard

Most of the mothers cried when they called to set up an interview appointment with me. They wanted to be heard, but the pain of the telling was palpable even in the initial contact we had on the telephone. We all have an innate need to be heard and validated. I believe these women wanted to be interviewed because they desperately wanted someone to hear them, someone who would listen without judgment. They had not felt that anyone would or could understand and care.

Featherstone (1980) wrote that "[mothers] looking for diagnoses are frightened and immensely vulnerable. They have already suffered days, months, even years, of agonizing doubt. They stand exposed and powerless before the experts. Indifference, condescension, or equivocation wounds them deeply" (p. 38). Mothers may perceive health care providers as judgmental and confrontational. One woman in the study feared prosecution and was concerned that I was from social services. Although she badly wanted to be heard and understood, it took time to get to the point where she was comfortable sharing. This speaks to the need to provide care and support within our health care, social services, and educational systems that is client-centered. The professionals working with mothers of children with FASD must examine their own biases and preconceptions so they can approach the women openly and non-judgmentally. We must be respectful of the dignity and worth of these women. It goes beyond clinical expertise to the need to develop relationships based on an understanding of who the woman is, what she is feeling, and what she needs to move forward to help herself and her child.

Women in my study wanted to have a non-judgmental person with whom they could share about their journey with the FASD diagnosis. They also wanted to share their stories because in so doing, they felt they could help other mothers. This was not part of the experience of receiving a diagnosis, but was a consistent message these women wanted me to take away from our interviews. Several of the mothers spoke of feeling empowered by sharing about themselves with me or in support groups. They wanted to protect others' children in a way they couldn't or didn't protect their own child. One study participant expressed the feelings of these mothers when she said "we can be a change for this in the future."

Women's Drinking

Mothers of children with FASD need help and support to cope with guilt and with the fears of what the future might bring (United Nations, 2004). Critical to success would be an approach by heath care providers, educators, and social service professionals that is non-judgmental and reflective, and that recognizes the strengths of the mothers and includes them in a partnered relationship.

Women drink for a number of reasons. Often they are shamed by their drinking but have no other means of coping with past and current stress. They carry this shame with them in whatever they do, including into the diagnostic process. The shame is then multiplied when they discover what they have done to their child. With no coping strategies, women continue to drink. Understanding a mother's thinking and reactions to the diagnosis of her child is critical. Does she deny the diagnosis or blame others for her use? Does she become depressed and shut down in her communications? Is she ready to begin the hard work of confronting her addictions? Where is she in her recovery? What sorts of support systems has she accessed or can she access? Exploring her reasons for drinking and her barriers to recovery will give clues to a client-centered approach that will ultimately prevent another birth of a child with FASD.

The Mother and the Diagnostic Process

The birth mother of a child diagnosed with FASD is dealing with her own sense of guilt and shame. She rightly or wrongly fears being judged just as harshly as she is judging herself. Her self-esteem is often low and she may be depressed. Mothers bear the burden of raising the child, and bear the blame if something goes wrong with that child (Dally, 1982). By understanding the experiences of the birth mother in receiving a diagnosis, including the part shame and self-judgment play in the diagnostic process, health care and educational specialists should be encouraged to think about how they approach their assessments and reports, including the words they use, the attitude they portray, and the time they give to mothers during the diagnostic process. They may need to take more time when they first begin to share their findings. They may want to be prepared to help the mother do the intense emotional work of processing and accepting the information, and be ready to offer resources for support and additional information.

Language that respects the mother and her child is critical. Mothers in my study felt stonewalled, summarily dismissed, discounted, and judged through the words and behaviors of the health care professionals who diagnosed their child. Words used carelessly, use of medical terminology when lay language would be more effective, minimization of the mother's concerns, disregard for how a diagnosis might impact her, and an appearance of being in a hurry (standing at the door versus sitting down) contribute to make a difficult meeting with the mother even more painful.

One of the primary reasons for undertaking this study was to consider the approach we take when we work with mothers during the diagnostic process. Typically, once a diagnosis is made by the team, a conference with the parents or caregivers is scheduled. The results of the assessment are shared by the team and planning begins for management of the many medical, social, and school problems of these very complex children. It is, after all, a child-focused process, a situation that is set up for the good of the child. Many times the team is ready to begin planning, but the mother may be reeling from the diagnosis. She may not be able to hear what is being said. The diagnostic protocols dominate the needs of the mother.

The desire is to get the services needed for the child as soon as possible, but when we are doing this are we disregarding the feelings and needs of the mother? Only when she is able to hear and accept the diagnosis can we begin the work that needs to happen for her and the child to be successful. Meaningful communication cannot happen if she is in the place where "it's all about her." She needs to be given time during the diagnostic meeting to do those first moments of grieving, to move beyond "I can't believe this is happening to me" and "what have I done" to a place of knowledge and acceptance needed to mother her child with FASD. We, the professionals, must avoid moving too fast to solutions. We must provide her time and resources to do her own emotional work on what the FASD label means to her and her child before we expect her to do the work needed for her child. By understanding the experiences of birth mothers on hearing the diagnosis of FASD, we as health care professionals and education specialists can create a more empathetic and effective diagnostic process that is mindful of their unique needs, fears, concerns, and challenges. This will ultimately lead to her being empowered and able to problem solve and contribute to the planning for her child.

I believe health care and educational specialists often create gaps in communication with the mothers with whom we work. According to Heffner (1978), we tend to interpret behavior either as a response to something *we* have done or as the result of someone else's inadequate personality or high-risk life situation. Depending on which interpretation we make, we may respond sympathetically or unsympathetically, with concern or with anger, with empathy and care or with indifference and haste. It is obvious that if our interpretations are incorrect, we are not responding to the other person at all but to our own perceptions. We are reacting out of our own sense of reality, rather than responding to the other person's reality. In effect, we are talking to ourselves while we think we are addressing someone else. Out of these failures of communication come the misunderstandings that lead to the breakdown of relationships. It is apparent that if a relationship is to function effectively, it becomes necessary for us to check out our perceptions against the other person's reality. Before responding we have to find out to what we are responding. Or, if we do respond, and our response creates a distance between us, we must consider the possibility that the assumptions on which we have been operating may not have been correct. It is my hope that in developing a more accurate understanding of birth mothers, we can understand how she is reacting to her child's diagnosis and can avoid creating gaps in communication that ultimately harm our relationship and do nothing to support the mother or help the child.

Traditionally, the relationship between a professional and a mother isn't typically a partnership working on behalf of the child. According to Heffner (1978), "professionals often behave as if they alone are advocates for the child; as if they are the guardians of the child's needs; as if the mother left to her own devices will surely damage the child, and only the professional can rescue him" (pp. 23-24). After all, the mother of a child with FASD has already proven she is capable of harming her child. This paternalistic stance places the mother in the position of a bad child, as well as a bad mother, and she becomes a person who is deserving of punishment. A mother's punishment is guilt. She is already experiencing this guilt knowing she is the cause of her child's difficulties. Being a good mother means doing what the professional says; after all, this person is the expert. Yet if she can't hear what the professional is saying because of her own emotions and needs, how can she follow through on the expectations that are being set? She then feels less effective, more at fault, and has increased guilt. The cycle of inadequate and inappropriate communication begins. It is the responsibility of the health professional to build an intentional relationship with the mother, by communicating consciously as part of building a trusting, mutually respectful, honest partnership. Communication includes both the giving and the receiving of information. Just as much as the mother is expected to use the wisdom of the health care or education team, she must also be appreciated as the expert on her child, and as an equal member of the team with valuable contributions that will improve the outcomes for her child.

Many of the women in my study shared the lack of validation they felt when reaching out for answers, and the judgment and lack of support they sensed after the words "Fetal Alcohol Spectrum Disorder" were spoken. Through the act of asking for help, a mother is often discredited about having any knowledge about her child (Heffner, 1978). A child with a problem is interpreted as having a mother with a problem. In the case of FASD, the mother may in fact continue to struggle with the alcohol use that caused the child's difficulties. She is most certainly dealing with her own pain, guilt, and shame. By listening to the story of the birth mother, health care providers or educational specialists can come to understand what the mother needs to know, and how fast she can hear it. It tells them how able she is to listen at just that point in time. Listening to the birth mother includes her as a member of the team in the diagnostic process. It also facilitates the team to meet her needs. Health care professionals want to fix people— that's why we're in this business. If we can't fix the problem, we have a tendency to look for a place to blame our failures. Mothers are handy targets for our frustration.

Every situation is different. Every diagnosis is different in how it manifests and what it means. Health professionals and educational specialists need to listen to each other, but more importantly, they need to listen to the mothers. In sharing the results of this study, I want professionals to know that they need to listen and they need to believe the mothers. They need to avoid biased thinking toward mothers and accept them as women who love their children deeply and want to do what's best for them.

Getting the Diagnosis Is the Same, Yet Different

One of the questions I kept coming back to as I listened to the birth mothers was, just how different is their experience from that of birth mothers whose children get any other kind of diagnosis? I was able to get glimpses of the experiences of those other mothers as I examined texts (such as Roskies' *Abnormality and Normality: The Mothering of Thalidomide Children*) that I was using to deepen my understanding of my research participants. I searched the literature with little success for first person accounts of experiences of mothers of children with diagnoses where the mothers might be deemed culpable. Then I stumbled across personal accounts by mothers of children with unspecified mental retardation (in *The Child Who Never* Grew) (Buck, 1950), autism spectrum disorder (in *A Slant of the Sun*) (Kephart, 1999), and learning disabilities (in *Reading David*) (Weinstein, 2003). In wrenching frankness these women exposed their perceived inadequacies as mothers. Their experiences were the same yet different from birth mothers of children with FASD.

Something doesn't seem right with my child. It seems that mothers intuit the subtleties and nuances of their child. This isn't unique to mothers of a child with FASD. Mothers seem to have a gut sense of their children and even when they cannot put words to it, they sense when something is wrong physically and emotionally.

The theme *I can't believe this is happening to me* is also not unique to FASD. It seems to be the first reaction to a child's diagnosis. The mother questions God, questions herself, and looks for reasons why she is being singled out and somehow punished.

It's when we get to the third theme, *I can't believe I've done this to my child,* which we begin to see both similarities and differences between birth mothers of children with FASD and birth mothers of children with other diagnosis. All of the mothers question what went wrong and look for a reason to understand what they might have done to their child. The difference is that mothers of children with FASD can readily identify the cause; they themselves were the damaging agent. Mothers of children with HIV/AIDS or genetic disorders feel the guilt, shame, and blame, but are better able to rationalize the fault. The intensity of the shame and guilt appears to be less at the core of who the mothers are in their mothering identities. Still other mothers are left wondering and looking for a reason; for these other mothers the self-blame is not in causing the difficulties, but in not recognizing and not intervening sooner. This may be another subtle difference between the shame and guilt experienced by the mothers of children with disabilities and those of children with FASD specifically. There is the guilt and shame, but there is also the not knowing where to hang those feelings—a more intense wondering felt by the mothers of children with other diagnoses—and the intensity of the guilt and shame of knowing you are the cause.

The theme *I need you to see me, hear me, help me* includes the fear of losing the child within the system. Mothers of children with disabilities fear that their child will fall through the cracks within complex medical and educational systems. Mothers of children with FASD share that fear, but they also fear losing the child to social services and the legal system. This theme also encompasses the need to be heard, respected by the professionals, and given the time and expertise needed to help their child. This need is felt by all mothers of children with disabilities, including FASD.

I can't fix it; I can't make it better. This theme is exemplified by worry about the future. All of the mothers worry about the future and the trials and difficulties their child will face. But there is a different sense to it. For birth mothers of children with FASD, there is a continuing sense of self-blame for a future gone bad. For them and for the other mothers, there is also a sense of not knowing and needing to protect their child. Birth mothers of children with FASD carry an added burden of knowing they are the source of their child's difficult life.

Understanding the Mothers

The purpose of the diagnosis is to help the mother help the child. A mother must be helped and empowered to find the best answers for herself and her child. She is the expert on her child, having watched the child from birth. She is the one who will know if the ideas being offered are going to be effective for her child in fact rather than in theory. By hearing the diagnosis, the mother has words for the problems her child is facing. She can now move forward to help her child. If the professionals work *with* her and not *for* her or in spite of her, she will be empowered. To do this, the professionals need to come to a shared understanding of what the diagnosis—the label--means to the mother and to her child.

The diagnosis or label doesn't have much value if we're trying to understand the mother and her lifeworld. Merleau-Ponty, Heidegger, Husserl, and Gadamer all hold the view that the person and her context need to be seen as a living whole. Our understanding of mothers "is always incomplete without taking into account their own understanding of themselves, their lived bodies, and the meaning that their life situations hold for them" (Dahlberg, K., Drew, N., & Nyström, M., 2001, p. 92).

I believe we live in a society that shames and blames mothers for the behaviors of their children or when something is "wrong" with the child. We want to explain the behavior or the disorder, and attach a cause to it, so that we can be assured it couldn't possible happen to me and my child. It happened to *that* mother of *that* child because the mother was bad somehow. If I can't find something to blame for the problems of that mother's child, I too am vulnerable to having a broken child. As a society, we sit in judgment. We judge to protect ourselves. In doing so, we distance ourselves. Because it doesn't involve me, I don't have to do anything about it. But as a society, we must embrace FASD as a preventable condition. We must understand that any woman, under the wrong circumstances, could give birth to a child with FASD. Women must be empowered to protect their children before they are even born, even as their means of protection isn't necessarily supported by society.

The mothers, too, can benefit from understanding about the mothering experience for others like her. She can come to realize that she is not unique in her shame and sadness. This understanding helps to normalize her feelings and thoughts, and it can change her self-perception of being bad and without redemption. She has made a mistake,

116

but she needs to go on. One of the study participants felt that all birth mothers should understand that "[FASD] is because of something that they did [to make] this happened, but they shouldn't blame themselves because you can't live your life like that. You made a mistake and hopefully you learned from it."

Mourning the Child Who Could Have Been

Universal to the mothers in this study, and to the mothers of children diagnosed with chronic and lifelong conditions, is a sense of guilt and blame. There is also a profound sorrow and a wish for things to be different. There is a mourning for the child who could have been. Mothers of children with disabilities grieve for the perfect child they have lost. What is this grieving process? Is it different for birth mothers of children with FASD?

> I think all parents who give birth to children with a disability must, at one time or another, wonder what their children would be like if they were not disabled. As we move through the phases of the cycle of loss—shock, anger, denial, grief, and eventual acceptance—at our own speed and periodically revisit one or more of these phases from time to time, we mourn the loss of the child we anticipated who suddenly vanished from our lives, the child who slipped through our hands before we had a chance to know him or her, the one who quietly disappeared into the crowd, never to be found. This mourning process, which I imagine to be similar to experiencing a miscarriage or the premature death of a child, is a necessary step before we can move on and begin to accept our disabled children into our lives. (Carter, 2004, p. 182)

An unborn child is expected with great anticipation. Mothers dream of and plan for a perfect baby who will grow to do great and wonderful things. What is it like to have those dreams shattered by a disability? How does a mother grieve? Grief can be conceptualized as a cognitive, behavioral, and emotional reaction to loss (Godress, Ozgul, Owen, & Foley-Evans, 2005). The mother has to deal with the loss of a "normal"

117

child and come to accept a different child (Paterson, 2002). She grieves for the loss of the person who could have been and the loss of her hopes, wishes, and aspirations. She grieves for the disruptions to her family and her relationships (Godress et al.). She must negotiate a new kind of mothering, deal differently with daily life than she had anticipated, and come to a point of compromise between accepting the disability and holding out hope for the disability to be taken away (Paterson). The grief is ongoing.

Kearney (2008) has differentiated two models of grief, time-bound and chronic. Time-bound grief, the predominate view, is depicted as a set of sequential stages through which a mother moves either toward acceptance of the disability or the neurosis of non-acceptance. From the perspective of chronic sorrow, a mother doesn't ultimately accept the disability; she comes to adapt to it in a functional sense. She continues to experience grief and sorrow over her lifetime, but she moves forward in life.

Models of time-bound grief are found in the work of Bright (1996), Kubler-Ross (1969), and Sen and Yurtsever (2007). These stages are reflected in the themes revealed in this study. Denial, the first emotional reaction is experienced when the mother first hears the diagnostic label. She is in shock. Her perfect child is not to be. Even though she may have suspected something was not quite right with her child, having the words said aloud makes her fears real. In her denial, she feels alone and singled out, afraid of the unknown, and full of guilt and shame for what she might have done to cause the disability. She wonders how she will handle the unanticipated responsibilities of her child's future. As she moves through this stage, she replaces her denial ("this can't be happening to me") with partial acceptance ("this is it, I can't make it change, so now what?"). Anger follows denial. She rages at God ("why me") and at others. Bargaining, the third stage, is often done in secret as a pact between God and mother. When she realizes bargaining won't work, the mother moves into the fourth stage, depression. She comes to understand that the disability is life long and she cannot make that fact change; she is devoid of feelings. If she is able to work through her depression, she comes to accept both emotionally and intellectually that she will always be the mother of a child with disabilities. In this final stage of acceptance, she is able to adjust and re-set her expectations and understands and moves to solve problems. She now hopes for a sense of normality in an abnormal situation.

The stage models of grief imply that total acceptance is necessary for healthy adjustment. But isn't it acceptable to be sad and to continually grieve the child that could have been? Using the chronic model of grieving, Blaska (2000) and Godress et al. (2005) found that mothers experience a range of intense emotions across time. But there were also times that mothers felt free of those emotions. Emotions were triggered by different events, particularly when developmental milestones were missed, but these emotions lessened in intensity over time.

Regardless of whether one espouses a time-bound or a chronic model of grieving, the mother of a child with disabilities (including FASD) searches for meaning in her grief and creates narratives for her stress and pain (Fisher & Goodley, 2007). Initially, she places a high value on the diagnosis and medical expertise, seeking yet fearing the answers. There is a sense that something is wrong and that knowing is better than not knowing, followed by a hope for recovery and a return to normalcy. Once the diagnosis is confirmed and the moment of relief in knowing passes, the reality of the "foreverness" and unfixable nature of the disability becomes the prevalent narrative. A mother may question what normal means and may also question the motives of health professionals and education specialists as they present intervention options. As did several of the women in my study, she may perceive the environment as hostile to her child as well as judgmental of her. Her narrative may then become one of challenging others and of self-empowerment and agency. She comes to see herself as the mother of a child with disabilities and as an independent fighter for her child. Or she comes to see herself as the bad mother, one who is the victim of moral sanction. She becomes un-empowered. The mothers in my study presented at both ends of this continuum. Some felt victimized and fearful of the system; others wanted to stand up for themselves and for other mothers. A mother's narratives, however, are open to change and negotiation as she and her child move through life. Empathetic health care and education professionals are key to helping birth mothers of children with FASD navigate their stages of grief and develop empowering personal narratives.

Moving On

For many of the birth mothers with whom I spoke, there was relief in hearing the diagnosis (in spite of the shame and self-blame), yet there were many emotional overtones. FASD is a birth defect that could have been prevented. The emotional reactions of the mother at the time of diagnosis ranged from guilt and shame, to anger, to denial, and to acceptance. But there was always a sense of sadness. These reactions, while perfectly normal, can create barriers to recognizing problems and developing intervention plans.

One of the questions I continue to have is whether or not the birth mothers can move forward with their lives. If so, when does it happen? We as health care providers and education specialists must remember that the child is not the diagnosis—neither is the mother. The birth mother is not to be defined by her behaviors, even though that's how she is feeling. "Encouraging motherliness" (Dally, 1982, p. 326) is critical and best accomplished by understanding the mother and helping her understand how to move on with the diagnosis in hand. Two of the study participants summed up several of the mothers' sentiments when they said:

> What I'm realizing is [I need] to accept what I chose to do, not to minimize it, not to say its okay, but to accept what I did so I can move forward so that I can start being a better productive mother for my children and help them have the most normal productive life possible. I can't say if I fully have accepted because the way I look at accepting it is me totally dealing with all my feelings and shame as a birth mother and letting it go, and then knowing that I have accepted, okay, this is what's done and not feeling all that and moving forward.

> It's been just one thing after another needing to accept. His schooling, the parenting with him, the special needs that have to be met, and the special people that are involved and revolving in his life. All of that took a whole lot of acceptance. I needed to accept it all and if I didn't, I'd stay stuck and what's the point in staying stuck when you know it's there and something's got to be done about it.

Other Things That Should Happen

Although not directly derived from the analysis of my themes, the exploration of the experiences of the women in my study led me to consider other things that should happen for these mothers. I believe it is important to consider what appropriate emotional support is for the mother after she hears the diagnosis of FASD for her child. Too often

121

the emphasis is on what to do with the child. The mother is not ready for this level of planning. She is still reeling. What does she need immediately? What will she need in the coming days and weeks? Health care providers need to put supports in place for mothers who "not only get hit with a tsunami, but now they're barely treading water and sinking fast." This study participant goes on to say that "[health care providers] need to put a safety net in place, but a lot of counties don't have the manpower to do it. Especially the one thing that should be tried is to establish if the parent is still drinking. Even if they're not, I think news like this would be pretty scary in terms of relapse." She felt that there should be a spot check a couple days after the diagnosis is given, either by social services or via contact with schools (for older children). "You feel guilt so you drink to shut up your head which causes more guilt which causes…"

I was somewhat dismayed, though not surprised, that a couple of the mothers whom I interviewed had more than one affected child. Drinking is a family issue. There is a genetic vulnerability and an environmental context to drinking. Women are especially vulnerable to continued drinking because they have many barriers to health care and substance use intervention (Beckman, 1994; DHHS, 2006; United Nations, 2004). Except in rare instances, prenatal alcohol use is not a deliberate attempt on the part of the mother to hurt her baby. (An exception was the mother in my study who hoped that by drinking she would somehow miscarry the child she knew she had already damaged.) This fact is critical in prevention. A high risk target population for FASD prevention efforts is the woman who already has a child with FASD. Key to preventing second births of children with FASD is proper and early diagnosis of the first child, then understanding why the mother continues to drink and providing her the resources and support she needs to overcome the barriers.

Also key to FASD prevention is changing public policy around women who seek help, and developing intervention programs and methodologies that address the unique needs of women rather than trying to retrofit models designed for men (United Nations, 2004). Pragmatically, women need programs that recognize their need to be mothers first and foremost and appreciate the lifestyle that goes along with motherhood. For example, they cannot drop all of their responsibilities to participate in support groups that are often held during the times of day when mothers are most needed by their children (e.g., evenings). And they cannot attend programs that are in difficult-to-reach or dangerous places; transportation is often a barrier (Beckman, 1994). Women-oriented programs would provide a broad range of coordinated components, including prenatal care, medical care, parenting education and the development of parenting skills, and training to develop self-esteem and coping skills (United Nations). Women need programs that provide mentorship from other women who have walked in their shoes (Beckman; Finkelstein, 1996). Women prefer getting support in group or social settings. Women-only support groups would help women accurately interpret and mediate events around them and develop effective responses (Beckman; Finkelstein). The phenomenon of women drinking (understanding why she continues to drink and what contributes to recovery), is an area for further research.

The fear of "the system" and the sense of being judged that was expressed by the mothers in my study also speak to our public policies that are, for the most part, disrespectful of and often punitive toward women. Reid, Greaves, and Poole (2008) wrote about mothers "trying to do good in a system and society that does not value or assist them" (p. 231). The women in my study spoke of a lack of power, and a sense of aloneness in a system that is not set up to help them. Their experiences reflect the literature on the provision of services to women. Women lose their individuality in a social system that is overloaded and under-funded. They become part of the system, mere case numbers in a case load of a social services representative who has time only to identify the women's faults so they can best direct their limited resources. Strengths go unrecognized and under-utilized. Women fall through the cracks. Women who seek services risk being identified and labeled as "high risk." The consequences of that label are significant; the mother risks losing her child, a fear expressed by a couple of the women in my study. In a system set up to protect the rights of children, resources shift away from the mother (who could use them for the support she needs to be a better mother) to a foster system or to significant others (Reid, Greaves, & Poole). The mother is punished for seeking resources, even though our social system and our society assigned responsibility to women—to mothers—to care for their children and families.

Considerations of the Study

The uniqueness of FASD is that the cause of the disabilities in a child can be directly linked to the mother's behavior. Except for some instances of HIV/AIDS and the use of tobacco and other drugs during pregnancy, no other diseases or disabilities share that characteristic. With tobacco and other drug use, the outcomes for the child can be ameliorated to a great extent if the child receives early intervention services. And with

HIV/AIDS, the mother is also sick; this creates a different set of dynamics. Studies that have addressed mothers' experiences of being culpable in their child's disability (HIV/AIDS, X-linked genetic conditions, FASD) have been limited to semi-structured interviews and surveys. There may be several reasons for this. Birth mothers may be reluctant—or are assumed to be reluctant—to share their experiences. Birth mothers are also difficult to locate. Many children diagnosed with FASD are in custodial care or have been adopted. Health care personnel may be struggling with their own biases (or their own behaviors) making the question a personally difficult one to ask. They also may assume they know the answers so the question is not a valid one to ask. Whatever the reason, to my knowledge, no other studies have been done that use a phenomenological approach to reflect on the lived experience of birth mothers receiving the diagnosis of FASD for their child. As with any phenomenological approach, the themes that I found are unique to the nine women whom I interviewed. A similar study might reveal the same themes, variations on these themes, and maybe even new ones. It would seem worthwhile to continue this question and this methodology to further understand the birth mothers who receive the FASD diagnosis for their child.

For this study, no attempt was made to selectively include or exclude mothers from being interviewed. In so doing, a number of new questions emerged. Is there a difference in the experience of mothers who receive the diagnosis at birth versus those who received that diagnosis when the child was older? Does it make a difference if the mother initiates the diagnostic process or if it comes from someone else? Does it make a difference if the study participant was or was not in recovery at the time of the diagnosis or at the time of the interview? What about whether or not the mother maintains custody of her child, has given up her child voluntarily to adoption or foster care, or has been forced to relinquish custody? Does that change her experience? Are there cultural or societal factors in how a mother experiences the diagnosis? Does socioeconomic status change perceptions of self, or perceptions of others toward the birth mother? Does it matter how the diagnosis is given or by whom? How is the concept of labeling itself perceived by mothers and how does that perception compare to that of health professionals? Do mothers question their ability to parent based on the meaning of the diagnosis or their own contribution to the child's disability? Is there ever a change in how mothers perceive themselves (e.g., how long do they carry the shame, guilt, and sense of badness)? What are the attitudes of foster or adoptive parents toward the birth mother? What are the attitudes of birth fathers toward the mothers or the children? How do the fathers parent these difficult children? How do health professionals experience giving the diagnosis?

I leave this study a more humble person. I have received the gift of stories shared freely by birth mothers who trusted me with their pain. I have gained respect for the struggles of women against their own self-judgments and the judgments of others as they try to do what is best for their children. I more deeply appreciate the deep sorrow of being the cause of a child's lifelong struggles. I more clearly appreciate the importance of understanding the truths about birth mothers—the alcohol abuse, addiction and recovery, or simply the mistakes made and the bad timing of the social drinker. It is my hope that sharing this understanding will lead other health care professionals and educational specialists to ask questions and listen to stories rather than shame, blame, and give pat

answers.

I would like to conclude this paper with two stanzas taken from the poem *Advice to Professionals Who Must Conference Cases.*

> If you could see the depth of this wrenching pain.
> If you could see the depth of our sadness
> then you would be moved to return
> our almost five-year-old son
> who sparkles in the sunlight despite his faulty neurons.
> Please give me back my son
> undamaged and untouched by your labels, test results
> descriptions and categories.
>
> If you can't, if you truly cannot give us back our son
> Then just be with us quietly,
> gently and compassionately as we feel.
>   (Fialka, 1997, p. 17).

References

Abel, E.I. (1995). An update on incidence of FAS: FAS is not an equal opportunity birth defect. *Neurotoxicology and Teratology, 17,* 437-443.

Abel, E.I. (1990). *Fetal alcohol syndrome.* Oradell, NJ: Medical Economics Books.

Anaisnais (n.d.). *Flutterings.* Retrieved June 23, 2009 from http://www.redbubble.com/people/anaisnais/writing/1636890-flutterings

Banis, S., Suurmeijer, Th.P.B.M., & van Peer, D.R. (1999). Child-rearing practices toward children with hemophilia: The relative importance of clinical characteristics and parental emotional reactions. *Family Relations, 48*(2), 207-213.

Barnard, K.E., & Martell, L.K. (1995). Mothering. In M.H. Bornstein (Ed.). *Handbook of parenting, vol. 3. Status and social conditions of parenting* (pp. 3-26). Hove, UK: National Institute of Child Health and Human Development.

Barr, H.M., & Streissguth, A.P. (2001). Identifying maternal self-reported alcohol use associated with fetal alcohol spectrum disorders. *Alcoholism: Clinical and Experimental Research, 25*(2), 283-287.

Beckman, L.J. (1994). Treatment needs of women with alcohol problems. *Alcohol Health and Research World, 18*(3), 206-211.

Blaska, J.K. (2000). *Cyclical grieving: Reoccurring emotions experienced by parents who have children with disabilities.* St. Cloud, MN: St. Cloud State University, Department of Child and Family Studies.

Bright, C. (Director) & Moore, A. (Editor). (1996). *Families of young children with special needs: Family crisis.* [Video]. Irvine, CA: Concept Media.

Brown, S. & Small, R. (1997). Being a 'good mother'. *Journal of Reproductive and Infant Psychology, 15*(2), 185-199.

Buchman, D. (2006). First you crawl. *Good Housekeeping, 242*(3), 1243-148.

Buck, P.S. (1950). *The child who never grew.* New York: John Day.

Bunting, S.M. (1996). Sources of stigma associated with women with HIV. *Advances in Nursing Science, 19*(2), 63-73.

Carter, S. (2004). For just one day. *Rehabilitation Counseling Bulletin, 47*(3), 181-183.

Center for Disease Control (1993). Fetal alcohol syndrome—United States. *Morbidity and Mortality Weekly Report, 42*, 339-341.

Center for Disease Control (2005). *U.S. Surgeon General releases advisory on alcohol use in pregnancy.* Retrieved July 26, 2007 from http://www.cdc.gov/ncbddd/fas/

Cogan, J. (2006). The phenomenological reduction. *The Internet Encyclopedia of Philosophy.* Retrieved September 27, 2008 from http://www.iep.utm.edu/p/phen-red/htm

Dahlberg, K., Drew, N., & Nyström, M. (2001). *Reflective lifeworld research.* Lund, Sweden: Studentlitteratur.

Dally, A. (1982). *Inventing motherhood: The consequences of the ideal.* New York: Schocken.

Department of Health and Human Services (2004a). *Gender differences in substance dependence and abuse.* Retrieved August 10, 2008, from http://oas.samhsa.gov/2k4/genderDependence/genderDependence.htm

Department of Health and Human Services (DHHS) (2004b). *Recovering hope: Mothers speak out about fetal alcohol spectrum disorders* [video]. (Available from the Substance Abuse and Mental Health Services Administration, Center for Substance Abuse Prevention, P.O. Box 2345, Rockville, MD 20847-2345).

Department of Health and Human Services (2004c, March 25). *Substance use among pregnant women during 1999 and 2000.* Retrieved August 8, 2008, from http://oas.samhsa.gov/2k2/preg/preg.htm

Department of Health and Human Services. (2006). *Substance abuse and dependence among women.* Retrieved August 8, 2008, from http://www.oas.samhsa.gov/2k5/women/women.htm

Dougherty, C., Brown, K., Pinch, W., Allegretti, J., Edwards, B., & McCarthy, V. (1990). *Confidentiality and pediatric HIV: A Creighton research project.* Omaha, Nebraska: Creighton University, Center for the Study of Religion and Society.

Ebrahim, S.E., Luman, E.T., Floyd, R.L., Murphy, C.C., Bennett, E. M., & Boyle, C. A. (1998). Alcohol consumption by pregnant women in the United States during 1988-1995. *Obstetrics and Gynecology, 92,* 187-192.

Elkins, M.J. (1991). Facing the gorgon: Good and bad mothers in the late novels of Margaret Drabble. In B.O. Daly & M. T. Reddy (Eds.), *Narrating mothers:*

Theorizing maternal subjectivities (pp. 111-124). Knoxville: University of Tennessee.

Featherstone, H. (1980). *A difference in the family: Life with a disabled child.* New York: Basic.

Fialka, J. (1997). *It Matters: Lessons from my son.* Toronto, ON: Illusion Press International.

Fink, E. (1972). What does the phenomenology of Edmund Husserl want to accomplish? In E. Fink, *Research in Phenomenology.* (A. Grugan, Trans.), (pp. 5-27). The Hague, Netherlands: Martinus Nijhoff. (Original work published 1966)

Finkelstein, N. (1996). Treatment programming for alcohol and drug dependent women. *The International Journal of Addictions, 28,* 1275-1309.

Fisher, P. & Goodley, D. (2007). The linear medical model of disability: Mothers of disabled babies resist with counter-narratives. *Sociology of Health and Illness, 29*(1), 66-81.

Fletcher, K. (2008). *Angels danced.* Retrieved February 9, 2009 from http:// www.mofas.org

Francis-Connelly, E. (2004). Mothering across the lifecourse. In S.A. Esdaile & J.A. Olson (Eds.), *Mothering occupations: Challenge, agency, and participation* (pp. 153-171). Philadelphia: F.A. Davis.

Gadamer, H.G. (1976). *Philosophical hermaneutics.* (D.E. Linge, Trans.). Los Angeles: University of California.

Gadamer, H.G. (1975). *Truth and method.* (Sheed & Ward Ltd., Trans.). New York: Seabury. (Original work published 1960)

Giorgi, A. (1997). The theory, practice, and evaluation of the phenomenological method as a qualitative research procedure. *Journal of Phenomenological Psychology, 28*(2), 235-260.

Godress, J., Ozgul, S., Owen, C., & Foley-Evans, L. (2005). Grief experiences of parents whose children suffer from mental illness. *Australian and New Zealand Journal of Psychiatry, 39,* 88-94.

Heffner, E. (1978). *Mothering: The emotional experience of motherhood after Freud and feminism.* Garden City, NY: Doubleday.

Heidegger, M. (1962). *Being and time.* (J. Macquarrie & E. Robinson, Trans.). San Francisco: Harper. (Original work published 1927)

Husserl, E. (1931). *Ideas: General introduction to pure phenomenology.* (W.R. Boyce Gibson, Trans.). New York: MacMillan. (Original work published 1913)

Husserl, E. (1964). *The idea of phenomenology.* (W.P. Alston & G. Nakhnikian, Trans.). The Hague, Netherlands: Martinus Nijhoff. (Original work published 1907)

Ingram, D. & Hutchinson, S.A. (1998). HIV-positive mothers and stigma. *Health Care for Women International, 20,* 93-103.

James, C.A., Hadley, D.W., Holtzman, N.A., & Winkelstein, J.A. (2006). How does the mode of inheritance of a genetic condition influence families? A study of guilt, blame, stigma, and understanding of inheritance and reproductive risks in familes with X-linked and autosomal recessive diseases. *Genetics in Medicine, 8*(4), 234-242.

Jones, K.L., & Smith, D.W. (1973). Recognition of the fetal alcohol syndrome in early infancy. *Lancet*, 999-1001.

Jones, K.L., Smith, D.W., Ulleland, C.N., & Streissguth, A.P. (1973). Pattern of malformation in offspring of chronic alcoholic mothers. *Lancet*, 1267-1271.

Kephart, B. (1999). *A slant of the sun: One child's courage.* New York: W.W. Norton.

Kearney, P. (2008). *Grief in the family context: Chronic grief (or is it periodic grief?).* Retrieved March 4, 2009 from

http://www.indiana.edu/~famlygrf/units/chronic.html

Klein, S.D. (1993). The challenge of communicating with parents. *Developmental and behavioral pediatrics, 14*(3), 184-190.

Kubler-Ross, E. (1969). *On death and dying.* New York: MacMillan.

Kulp, J. (2008). *Withered.* Retrieved July 7, 2009 from

http://www.authorsden.com/visit/viewpoetry.asp?AuthorID=80097&id=224986

Kvale, S. (1996). Hermeneutical canons of interpretation. In *Interviews: An introduction to qualitative research interviewing* (pp. 48-50). Thousand Oaks, CA: Sage.

LaFever, L.B. (2000). *Cheers! Here's to the baby!* Seattle: Crawford.

LaFever, L. (Winter, 1995). Help, hope and healing from the inside out. *F.A.S. Times*, Tacoma, WA: FAS/FRI Publications. Retrieved June 19, 2007 from

http://www.fetalalcoholsyndrome.ort/sister1.txt

Larson, E.A. (2000). Mothering: Letting go of the past ideal and valuing the real. *American Journal of Occupational Therapy, 54*(3), 249-251.

Lazarre, J. (1976). *The mother knot.* Boston: Beacon.

Leavitt, C. (2006). Learning mother love. *Psychology Today, 39*(4), 44-45.

Lupton, C., Burd, L., & Harwood, R. (2004). Cost of fetal alcohol spectrum disorders. *American Journal of Medical Genetics, 127C*(1), 42-50.

Madden, N.A., Terrizzi, J., & Friedman, S.B. (1982). Psychological issues in mothers of children with hemophilia. *Developmental and Behavioral Pediatrics, 3*(3), 136-142.

Madison, G.B. (1988). The hermeneutics of postmodernity: Figures and themes. In J.M. Edie (Ed.). *Studies in phenomenology and existential philosophy* (pp. 28-31). Bloomington: Indiana University Press.

Marsh, D.B. (Ed.) (1995). *From the heart: On being the mother of a child with special needs.* Bethesda, MD: Woodbine.

Marshall, H. (1991). The social construction of motherhood: An analysis of childcare and parenting manuals. In A. Phoenix, A. Woollett, & E. Lloyd, (Eds). *Motherhood: Meanings, practices and ideologies,* (pp. 13-27). Newbury Park, CA: Sage.

May, P.A. & Gossage, J.P. (2001). Estimating the prevalence of fetal alcohol syndrome: A summary. *Alcohol Research and Health, 25*, 159-167.

Mayers, A.M., Naples, N.A., & Nilson, R.D. (2005). Existential issues and coping: A qualitative study of low-income women with HIV. *Psychology and Health, 20*(1), 93-113.

McKinney, V. (Spring, 1998). Nature vs nurture. *F.A.S. Times,* Tacoma, WA: FAS/FRI
    Publications.

Merleau-Ponty, M. (1962). *Phenomenology of perception.* (C. Smith, Trans.). New York:
    The Humanities Press. (Original work published 1945)

Merleau-Ponty, M. (1968). *The visible and the invisible.* (A. Lingis, Trans.). Evanston:
    Northwestern University Press. (Original work published 1964)

Miles, M., Burchinal, P., Holditch-Davis, D., Wasilewski, Y., & Christian, B. (1997).
    Personal, family, and health-related correlates of depressive symptoms in mothers
    with HIV. *Journal of Family Psychology, 11*(1), 23-34.

National Council on Alcoholism and Drug Dependence (2002). *Use of alcohol and other
    drugs among women.* Retrieved July 27, 2007 from
    http://www.ncadd.org/facts/women.html

Ostrom, R.A., Serovich, J.M., Lim, J.Y., & Mason, T.L. (2006). The role of stigma in
    reasons for HIV disclosure and non-disclosure to children. *AIDS Care, 18*(1), 60-
    65.

Oxford English Dictionary (2006). Retrieved July 27, 2007 from
    http://dictionaryoed.com.floyd.lib.umn.edu

Paterson, B. (2002). Review: Mothers of children with physical and mental disabilities
    experience emotional compromise between acceptance and denial. *Qualitative
    Health Research, 12*(4), 515-530.

Phoenix, A. & Woollett, A. (1991). Motherhood: Social construction, politics, and

135

psychology. In A. Phoenix, A. Woollett, & E. Lloyd, (Eds). *Motherhood: Meanings, practices and ideologies,* (pp. 13-27). Newbury Park, CA: Sage.

Polkinghorne, D. (1989). Phenomenological research methods. In R.S. Valle & S. Halling (Eds.), *Existential-phenomenological perspectives in psychology: Exploring the breadth of human experience.* (pp. 41-60). New York: Plenum.

Randall, R. (Executive Producer) & Ackerman, R.A. (Director). (1994). *David's mother* [Motion picture]. United States: Hearst Entertainment, Inc. & Morgan Hills Films.

Reid, C., Greaves, L., & Poole, N. (2008). Good, bad, thwarted or addicted? Discourses of substance-using mothers. *Critical Social Policy, 28,* 211-234.

Reed, B. G. (1987). Developing women-sensitive drug dependence treatment services: Why so difficult? *Journal of Psychoactive Drugs, 19*(2), 151-164.

Roskies, E. (1972). *Abnormality and normality: The mothering of thalidomide children.* Ithaca, NY: Cornell University Press.

Scott, A. (2003). *Husserl's ideas on a pure phenomenology and on a phenomenological philosophy.* Retrieved September 27, 2008 from http://www.angelfire.com/md2/timewarp/husserl.html

Sen, E. & Yurtsever, S. (2007). Difficulties experienced by families with disabled children. *Journal of the Society of Pediatric Nurses, 12*(4), 238-252.

Streissguth, A.P. (1997). *Fetal alcohol syndrome: A guide for families and communities.* Baltimore: Paul H. Brooks.

Streissguth, A.P. & O'Malley, K. (2000). Neuropsychiatric implications and long-term consequences of fetal alcohol spectrum disorders. *Seminars in Clinical Neuropsychiatry, 5*(3), 177-190.

United Nations (2004). *Substance abuse treatment and care for women: Case studies and lesions learned.* Vienna: Smithers Foundation.

van Manen, M. (2002). *Inquiry: Epistemology of practice.* Retrieved June 12, 2007 and September 27, 2008 from http://phenomenologyonline.com

van Manen, M. (1997). *Researching lived experience: Human science for an action sensitive pedagogy.* Toronto, Ontario: Transcontinental.

Wallner, A. (Winter, 2002/Spring, 2003). Another year of crises and choices. *F.A.S. Times,* Tacoma, WA: FAS/FRI Publications.

Weinsheimer, J.C. (1985). *Gadamer's hermeneutics: A reading of truth and method.* New Haven: Yale University.

Weinstein, L. (2003). *Reading David.* New York: Berkley.

Appendix A

CONSENT FORM
Diagnosing the Child, Diagnosing the Mother:
The Lived Experience of Birth mothers of Children with FASD

You are invited to be in a research study that will look at the experience of birth mothers when they find out there children have Fetal Alcohol Spectrum Disorder (FASD). You were chosen as a possible participant because you have recently been given an FASD diagnosis for your child. I ask that you read this form and ask any questions you may have before agreeing to be in the study.

I am Diane Anderson, an occupational therapist on FASD diagnostic teams and a graduate student in Family, Youth and Community Education within the College of Education at the University of Minnesota. I will be doing this study.

Background Information
The reason for doing this study is to find out more about what it is like for you personally to find out your child has FASD.

Procedures:
If you agree to be in this study, you will be asked to do the following things: take part in an interview that will take about 1½ -2 hour. The interview will be tape recorded and what you say will also be written down to make sure I am getting the information accurately. You might be asked for a short follow-up interview to make sure your experience is clearly understood. Once the interviews from all of the moms that are in the study have been read and I have written a summary of what everyone has said, you will be able to read the summary and give me any additional thoughts you have about what has been written or about your experience. I am doing this to make sure that I completely and accurately understand your experience.

Risks and Benefits of the Study
The study has two risks. First, finding out that your child has FASD may be upsetting to you, and the interview questions may ask you to describe hard and painful feelings and experiences. Second, because you are being asked to share your personal information, you may consider the questions an invasion of privacy. You may share only the information you are comfortable sharing, and you may ask to stop the interview at any time by saying "I don't want to do this."

A benefit to doing the interviews for you personally is that you have a chance to share feelings about your child's FASD diagnosis and what it means to you. There are no direct benefits to the study participants.

Compensation:
To thank you for giving me some of your valuable time, you will receive a $20 gift card following the first interview, and a $10 gift card for participating in the follow-up interview if that is necessary.

Confidentiality:
The records of this study will be kept private. I will share the information from the interviews only with classmates and a professor in the class I am taking to learn how to do good interviews. There will be no information shared that would let anybody identify you. In any sort of report I might publish, I will not include any information that will make it possible to identify you. Research records will be locked in a safe place and only I will have access to the records. I will transcribe the tape recordings into written form and the tapes will be erased.

Voluntary Nature of the Study:
Being a participant in this study is voluntary. Your decision whether or not to take part in this study will not affect your current or future relations with the University of Minnesota or the diagnostic clinic where you got the FASD diagnosis for your child. If you decide to participate, you are free to not answer any question or stop at any time without affecting those relationships.

Contacts and Questions:
My name is Diane Anderson and I am running this study. You may ask any questions you have now. If you have questions later, **you are encouraged** to contact me at The College of St. Scholastica, Occupational Therapy Department, 218-723-5915 (or email at danders4@css.edu). You may also call my advisor Dr. Jane Plihal in the College of Education and Human Development, 612-624-3069.

If you have any questions or concerns about this study and would like to talk to someone other than me or my advisor, **you are encouraged** to contact the Research Subjects' Advocate Line, D528 Mayo, 420 Delaware St. Southeast, Minneapolis, Minnesota 55455; (612) 625-1650.

You will be given a copy of this information to keep for your records.

Statement of Consent:
I have read the above information. I have asked questions and have received answers. I consent to participate in the study.

Signature:_____ Date: _____

Signature of Investigator:_____ Date: _____

Appendix B

Interview 4	Thematic aspects	Possible thematic statements
So you're just starting to understand about what fetal alcohol is, and you're just starting to understand that it's cuz you drank, and....what is that? Knowing that...		
very, very guilty. And very...like, what was I thinking. How could I possibly have done that to my child? I've got a lot of guilt behind it. I guess, I guess that's part of my unfitness as a parent. I don't know how to try to, ah...I know my sister tells me I can never make up or try to compensate and help my child in every way that I can to...not overcome it, but be able to not let it be like a crutch or something.	Guilt Unfit mother Advise from sister-- sharing	Unfitness – what have I done?
What does it mean to be a fit mom? You said that a couple times. Things like, I need to be a fit mom. Um, I need to be the kind of mom he needs. I need to be a good mom. What does that mean for you as a mom with a kid with fetal alcohol syndrome?		
Well, I guess it would mean that, um, I would be able to role model certain situations that I read about. I would be able to understand why certain things are not appropriate. Ah, meet all his basic needs – food, clothing, shelter. I manage to do that to a certain extent, but like, I...ah...I struggle with trying to keep food in the house. Keep him in clothes-both winter, summer, fall. And , ah....just be a better mom. I don't...I have ideas of what that means. It's just kind of hard to put into words right now. (long pause) I guess maybe I should be more involved in his school, his education. I am, but I feel like I'm at a...ah...a stumbling block.	Getting the dx means not being a fit mom – not understanding the dx, not meeting needs	What can I do differently? How can I make it better?

Interview 3	Thematic aspects	Possible thematic statements
If I can be the myth buster, cuz nobody would expect it from me. I can pass myself off as this, this competent together person. Because I am. So then it blows up in people's face a little bit. So then, maybe it'll wake some people up. Like, oh, and you're telling people? You're admitting that? It's like, well, yeah. How can people not do this to other children if they don't know? So it'll be, so yeah, that's the compulsion piece. I just hate, hate status quo when it's hurting people. When it's hurting people. So I like to, to take a stand. I'm somebody who likes to take a stand.	Telling others as a prevention thing	Disclosing to help others
The other thing you talked about is being validated.		
Validation is totally related to this last thing I was talking about. Um, about challenging the status quo. So to validate my experience as being real and true takes the blinders off. And there were people I was talking to face-to-face who wouldn't validate me. I have a piece of paper that said, yeah, now it's valid now. And so the diagnosis gave validity to what I knew to be true. So after being disregarded the validation was important. And it will also validate other women with experiences as they disclose. That whole team thing. You know, it's like I'm not the only one. The only college educated, white, middle class woman out there who...I brought some validation. So...past tense, present tense, future tense.	Feeling validated through disclosure

Value of diagnosis

Good labeling- bad labeling | Telling others

Labeling |
| *Your experience will bring them that validation?* | | |
| Because they won't feel alone. Because I don't have hang-ups about it. I think of...normalizing an experience. That can have shame to it, you know. And shame is not a good thing for women to feel about something that they may have been ignorant about or misinformed about by | Normalizing the experience can have shame to it as well

Ignorant health care | Varieties of shame – moving on from here.

How is this |

professionals. You know what I mean? You know the doctor told me it was OK. I'm going to go see him sometime, or write him a letter. I will. You know? Because it's like, you're wrong buddy.	professionals -	different re: feelings of shame?

Interview 6	Thematic aspects	Possible thematic statements
What I learned was the brain was always wanting to go go go, so, I kinda knew something in my heart, something's not right with him, and so I kept asking questions, how do I find out what the alcohol did to him? So when I was lucky enough to meet [ ] at one of the [ ] meetings, he said, we can't actually tell unless they have the physical facial features, or slow development in like speech or crawling or something. So like, actually, when [ ] was almost a year and a half, I got on the phone and made an, got an appointment for him to be diagnosed. I wanted to be on top of this, because I was worried about what I did to him, so I feel guilty.	Something's wrong Getting the diagnosis guilt	Something's not right with my baby I've done something bad to my child
Tell me more about that feeling guilty.		
It's an every day thing. It's like when he falls down and hurts himself, or when he breaks something, I know it's his brain, not, I shouldn't say not working right, but thinking different. He thinks different, but not that it doesn't work right, he just thinks different. So I have to deal with that guilt everyday. I have to like go to church a lot, and if it wasn't for these care givers meetings, I'd feel like I was all alone. You should tell some of the mothers that they should go. My guilt is a daily thing. I think I better go to therapy just to help myself deal with it. Cuz I've gotta like sweep all my feelings and my guilt under the carpet so I can deal with him, cuz he's really, he's intense, he's intense.	Guilt Feeling alone It effects me	All about me

When you talk about everyday, it's an everyday occurrence. Tell me more about that.		
If I knew I was pregnant, I wouldn't drink. God be it, I drank and I did it to him. I have to help him deal with his challenges. I don't want to say disabilities because it makes me feel guiltier. I want to say, I'm happy with challenges. He's gonna have challenges. He's gonna have challenges the rest of his life. He's so young right now, we don't know what areas he's gonna have these challenges	My fault

Guilt-have to move past to help child

Challenges that go on forever | What have I done to my child?

I can't make it go away |

Interview 7	Thematic aspects	Possible thematic statements
I feel pretty, um…(long pause)…discouraged about that? Because I don't know what the outcome is going to be with that kid. (Heavy sigh, tearful)	Don't know what the outcome will be	Sadness - forever
You said remorse earlier. And now you say discouraged.		
Both. I can't fix it. And I can't make it go away. (Long pause) And the additional damage he has done to himself based on, you know, secondary characteristics, or whether he would have been that way without prenatal alcohol exposure, I don't know. I really have unanswered questions, on the one hand about what would have been different. You know. And I don't need those answers. Nobody can change it anyway. You know. He can change his own future to a certain extent.	What would have been different? Lost potential, hopes, dreams

Other disabilities | It's forever; I can't fix it. |
| *You also mentioned integrity. That having a diagnosis now gives you…. more integrity.* | | |
| I think women are in denial about it, or they're secretive about their use. Or they use and they don't want to expose themselves. But we can't make this disability go away as long as we hide it. So, part of the movement forward to stop this is | We can't make this disability go away | Desire to prevent others from this experience. |

for people to say, you know what, it's all about service. So, you become one of the statistics. And then that makes the statistic more real. To people who don't want to believe the statistic. It's that whole thing that happens in the chemical dependency field. Is if you know, if you are chemically dependent, you have more credibility. Or if you struggled with depression, you're more credible, or whatever. You know? And so, so for me, I think it increases my credibility when I speak to women like me.	Becoming one of the statistics increases credibility	Opposite of wanting to hide it – protecting others in a way couldn't or didn't protect own child

0 1341 1485056 0

CPSIA information can be obtained at www.ICGtesting.com
Printed in the USA
LVOW020849021212

309746LV00005B/269/P

9 781243 725011